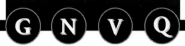

INTERMEDIATE

GNVQ

Health &
Social Care

SECOND EDITION

■ **HILARY THOMSON** ■ **CAROLINE HOLDEN** ■ **SYLVIA ASLANGUL**

Hodder & Stoughton

A MEMBER OF THE HODDER HEADLINE GROUP

Order queries: please contact Bookpoint Ltd, 39 Milton Park, Abingdon, Oxon OX14 4TD. Telephone: (44) 01235 400414, Fax: (44) 01235 400454. Lines are open from 9.00 – 6.00, Monday to Saturday, with a 24 hour message answering service. Email address: orders@bookpoint.co.uk

British Library Cataloguing in Publication Data
A catalogue record for this title is available from The British Library

ISBN 0 340 74314 X

Second edition 2000
First published 1998
Impression number   10 9 8 7 6 5 4 3 2 1
Year   2003 2002 2001 2000

Copyright © 2000

Cover photo from Photofusion.

Typeset by Multiplex Techniques Ltd, St Mary Cray, Kent.

Printed in Spain for Hodder & Stoughton Educational, a division of Hodder Headline Plc, 338 Euston Road, London NW1 3BH, by Graphycems.

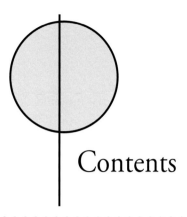

Contents

Acknowledgements   iv

Introduction   v

Learning to learn – A study skills guide   1

Chapter 1: Health, Social Care and Early Years Provision   54

Chapter 2: Promoting health and well-being   156

Chapter 3: Understanding personal development   233

Index   293

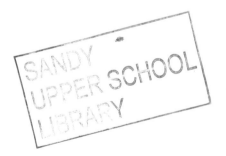

ACKNOWLEDGEMENTS

Thanks to the following for their valuable help:

Carolyn Meggitt for permission to adapt some of her material on child development; Sutton Carers Centre, the Weekend Break Project, Sutton Mencap, Sutton Bereavement Service for advice and information; Thomas Garrod for Fig. 1.36; Charlotte Dodwell's design for Fig. 1.38; Friends for the Young Deaf for Fig. 1.53; the Stonham Housing Association for permission to reproduce Tables 11/12 in the 'Learning to Learn' chapter from their publication 'Care Practice Manual for Supported Housing'; Jenny Cogan for permission to reproduce the figure 'The importance of reviewing' in the chapter 'Learning to Learn'; David Boyt for figures 2.1 and 2.4. The Back-up Trust for Fig. 2.14, showing Rob Smith and Dave Nash.

Thank you to our families for their help, support, and encouragement.

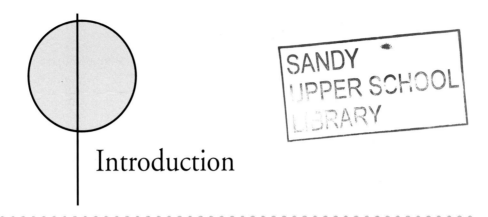

Introduction

The recent changes to GNVQ (**G**eneral **N**ational **V**ocational **Q**ualifications) courses have meant that completely new texts are required. This book covers, chapter by chapter, the three new Intermediate GNVQ Health and Social Care compulsory units. These units were set centrally and are the same irrespective of the awarding body offering the qualification (Edexcel, AQA and OCR – see end of this introduction for contact details). The compulsory units, and therefore this book, will help you to develop your understanding of health and social care, and will introduce you to some of the skills and knowledge you need to work in health and social care services.

STRUCTURE OF THE COURSE

The intermediate course consists of 3 compulsory units and 3 optional units.

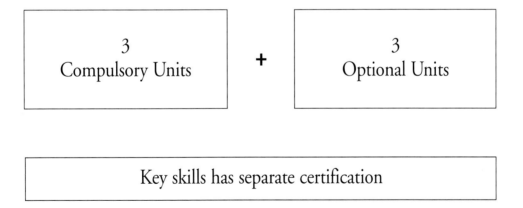

FIGURE 1 *Structure of the Intermediate Course.*

Taking an Intermediate GNVQ course is like doing four GCSEs in one year, at the standard grades A* to C. You may take one or two GCSEs alongside your GNVQ, or you may take extra GNVQ optional units or other qualifications.

ASSESSMENT

Each compulsory unit will receive a Pass, Merit, or Distinction and there will be an overall grade awarded for the whole qualification. Assessment will be through a combination of internal and external requirements.

The internal assessment, by which two thirds of the course will be assessed, will be through the marking of assignments by centres. There will be a standards moderation system to make sure that the grades given by centres are in line with national standards.

COMPULSORY UNITS	ASSESSMENT METHOD
1 Health, Social Care and Early Years Provision	External
2 Promoting Health and Well-Being	Internal
3 Understanding Personal Development	Internal

TABLE 1 *Unit assessment.*

KEY SKILLS

The remaining third of the course will be assessed through work externally set and marked by the awarding bodies. This will include either tests or externally set and marked assignments. Table 1 shows how each unit will be assessed. Each chapter ends with the type of assessment which will be used for the unit covered by that chapter.

KEY SKILL UNITS
• Application of number
• Communication
• Information Technology

TABLE 2 *Key Skill units.*

Key skills (Table 2) are general skills which are valued by employers, colleges and universities. They are an integral part of GNVQ qualifications. However, Key Skills will be separately certificated, and achievement of a GNVQ will not be dependent on achievement of Key Skills. It is possible to cover the key skills through the three compulsory units, and the activities give ample opportunities where you can develop Key Skills evidence.

Book content

The **first section** of the book focuses on the **study skills** which are essential to Intermediate GNVQ students. Students will find this an invaluable resource, particularly at the start of their course.

Unit 1 explores the **structure of health and social care and early years services**, and the main roles of the people who work within these services, as well as the skills that are needed for this work. Communication skills are very important and these are covered within the chapter. The care value base, which is linked to NVQs and underpins all the work in health and social care, is covered in detail, looking at aspects of discrimination, confidentiality and individual rights.

Unit 2 focuses on **Promoting Health and Well-being**. It starts with definitions of health and well-being, and how aspects of health and well-being differ between different people and groups of people. Factors which can have either positive or negative effects on health care are covered for example, diet, exercise, substance abuse, and socio-economic factors. There is information on Health Promotion, and advice given on how to provide others with information which will help them improve their health and well-being. An explanation is given on how to measure indicators of physical health, such as peak flow and pulse rate.

Unit 3 focuses on **Understanding personal development**. It starts with a description of the physical, social, intellectual and emotional growth that takes place from infancy through to old age. The social and economic factors which can affect development are considered. Self-concept is described, along with the factors it can be affected by such as age, culture and gender. Predictable and unpredictable life changes, and their positive and negative effects, are covered. The chapter concludes with the types of support available and details of how to identify the physical, emotional, intellectual and social needs of a person in order to provide appropriate support.

At the end of each chapter is:

- an explanation of **Key Words and Phrases**
- a **list of useful resources** (As well as written sources, these lists include helpful addresses, phone numbers and web sites.)
- An **example of a test or assignment**, depending on how the particular unit will be assessed (see Table 1).

What can I do with my Intermediate GNVQ?

Following the successful completion of your Intermediate Health and Social Care GNVQ, you might decide to:

- take an **Advanced GNVQ course**
- **start work** An Intermediate Health and Social Care GNVQ is a good basis for work in some areas of residential care, health care or community work. It can also lead to more specialised NVQs in care-related areas.

FINDING OUT MORE

Qualifications and Curriculum Authority (QCA), 29 Bolton Street, London W1Y 7PD
Web site: www.qca.org.uk/gnvq

Awarding bodies

- **EDEXCEL**   Tel: 020 7393 4444   Website: www.edexcel.org.uk
- **OCR**   Tel: 01203 470033   Website: www.ocr.org.uk
- **AQA**   Tel: 020 7294 2468   Website: www.aqa.org.uk

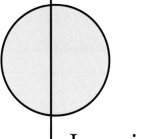

Learning to Learn – A Study Skills Guide

Students taking the Intermediate GNVQ in Health and Social Care will find that the course is designed with **two** purposes in mind. **One** is to enable students to gain knowledge and experience in the vocational area of health and social care and **the other** is to '**learn how to learn**' more effectively. Most students cope well with the new demands this course makes upon them. Others may need to investigate new ways to manage difficulties they have always experienced, perhaps because of a condition such as dyslexia or a disability. There are also certain people, such as older students returning to study after a break from education, who may encounter new problems. For **all** of us, however, **learning how to learn is essential for success**. The best results will be achieved by students who take the following advice to heart:

"Wise is she who knows when she does not know!"

This chapter has been written to help you answer the following questions:

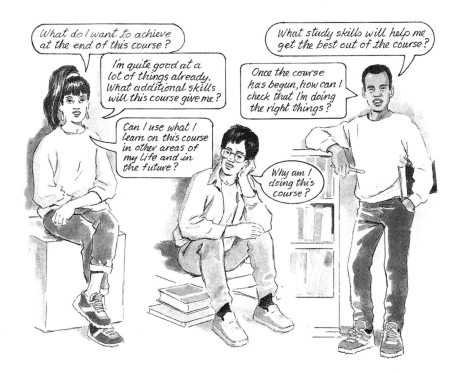

FIGURE 1 *Questions you should ask before beginning the course.*

This chapter covers:

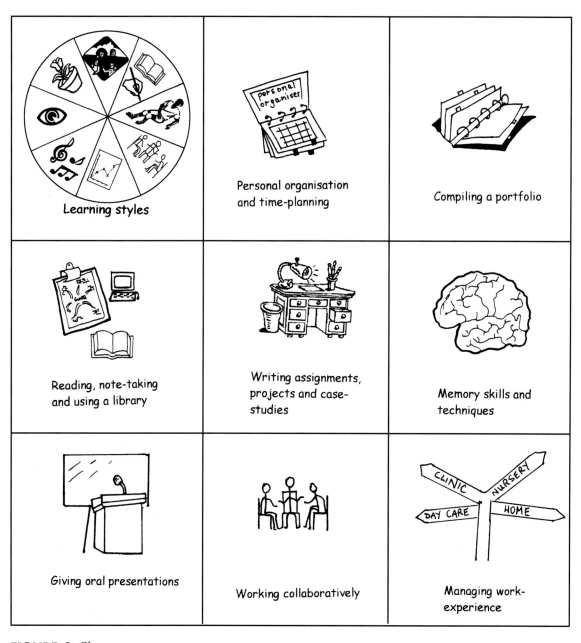

FIGURE 2 *Chapter content.*

Throughout the chapter there are activities to encourage you to investigate the strategies suggested. The chapter also offers support for the development of Key Skills. Key Skills are the general skills that can help you improve your own learning and performance. They are relevant to what you do in education and training, work, and life in general. Students taking this course will also be working towards gaining the Key Skills Qualification. This qualification recognises achievement in the three Key Skills units of **communication, application of number** and **information technology**. Because this chapter encourages you to focus on what you are learning and how you are learning, it will help you achieve the relevant aspects of each Key Skill. The chapter concludes with a **glossary** and a list of **useful resources**.

Learning styles

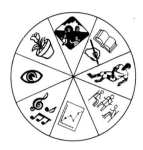

All of us learn in different ways. We each have a combination of different types of intelligence. While some people may be good 'all–rounders', able to learn, depending upon the task in hand, through a wide variety of methods, others may find it much easier to use just one or two 'learning styles'. A learning style is a way of learning information. For example, some people are organised and analytical. They make lists of what they have to do and plan their time carefully. Others do things when they occur to them, sometimes on the spur of the moment, often prompted by ideas they have been thinking about for a while. While some people learn best by listening and discussing things, other need to 'see' information visually, in pictures, diagrams and colours.

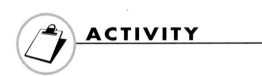

ACTIVITY

1   **What are your preferred learning styles? Use Figure 3 to think about the methods of working which best suit your learning styles. Make a note of these. You will need to keep these in mind as you read this chapter.**

2   **Are you an 'all-rounder' (with no strong preference for any particular way of working) or do you find certain methods of working easier than others?**

People working in health and social care do need good interpersonal and intrapersonal skills. It would not be surprising if students who choose to study this course felt they were 'strong' in these areas or wanted to develop these particular skills. However, while it may be that we will learn best through channels which work for us, there is nothing to stop us from exploring new ways to learn. The rest of this chapter contains many ideas for studying effectively and for developing competence in the wide range of academic and vocational skills required from students taking the Intermediate GNVQ in Health and Social Care.

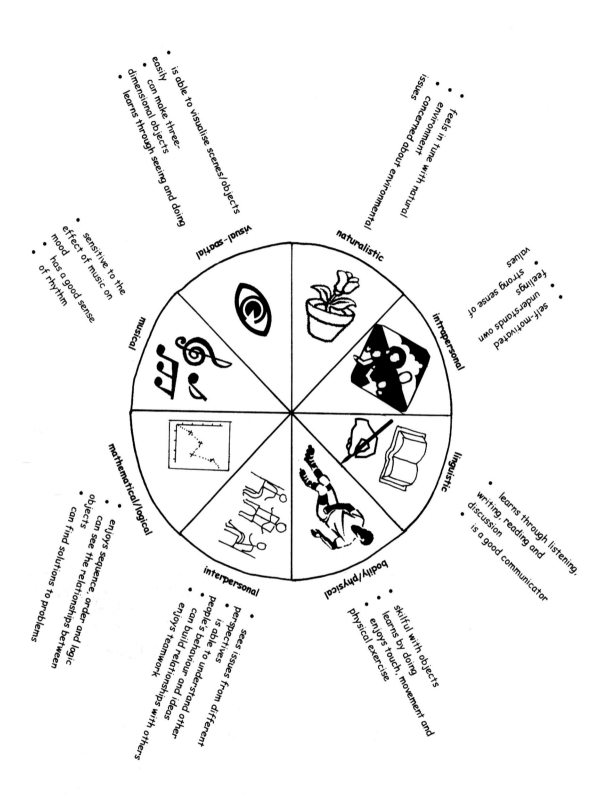

FIGURE 3 *Learning styles.*

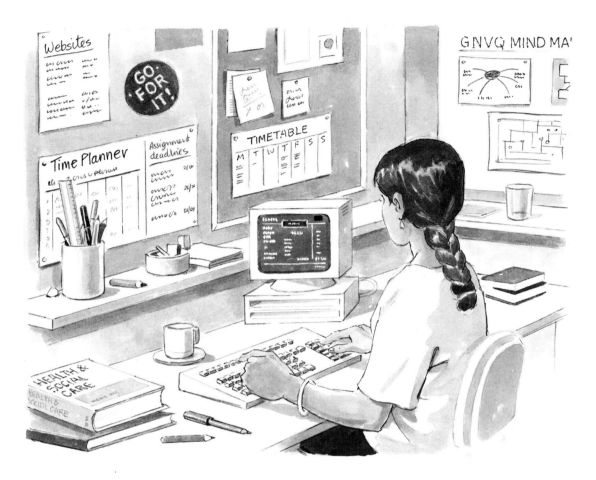

FIGURE 4 *Organising study periods.*

Personal organisation and time-planning

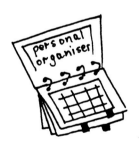

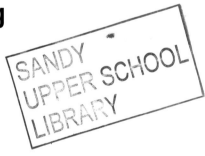

Virtually any activity (washing dishes, tidying your room, staring at the wall, fetching just *one more* small snack) can seem preferable to working on an assignment or settling down to revision. However, when work is postponed regularly, deadlines and examination dates can increase feelings of disorganisation and panic and can trigger a "flight" response. It can become tempting to produce the minimum work possible or event to abandon assignments completely. Excuses have to be invented, deadlines renegotiated, further assignments become due before the last ones are completed and before long the course begins to feel overwhelming and unmanageable.

Weekly Planner

	MONDAY	TUESDAY	WEDNESDAY	THURSDAY	FRIDAY	SATURDAY	SUNDAY
	Who can help?	Who can help?	Who can help?	Who can help?	Who can help?	Who can help?	Who can help?
	Best time to study?	Best time to study?	Best time to study?	Best time to study?	Best time to study?	Best time to study?	Best time to study?
morning	morning	morning	morning	morning	morning	morning	morning
afternoon	afternoon	afternoon	afternoon	afternoon	afternoon	afternoon	afternoon
evening	evening	evening	evening	evening	evening	evening	evening

TABLE 1 *Weekly Planner.*

Of course, people can have very good reasons for finding their workload difficult to manage: child care or other family responsibilities, the need to earn money through part-time work and unexpected traumas or illness, can all increase the pressure on students. However, if you are generally enjoying your course and finding the work stimulating and interesting, you are likely to want to find a way of organising your time so that you can keep a balance between your work, your social life and your other interests and commitments.

Planning time

There are only so many hours in a week. Although keeping rigidly to a **"Weekly Planner"** or timetable (such as the one in Table 1) will not always be easy or desirable, it should help you to focus on what free time you have in a week and which "chunks" of it can be used for course work and revision.

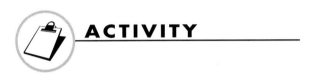 **ACTIVITY**

Photocopy and enlarge the planner on page 6 or draw up your own.

Now mark on:

- **Your college or school time tabled commitments, i.e. your lectures and lessons.**
- **Any paid work, housework or child care/family commitments.**
- **Travel times.**
- **Times you normally spend with friends/sports activities/other leisure pursuits**
- **Any 'unmissable' T.V. programmes (not too many!)**

What "chunks" of time have you left for studying?

- **In the day?**
- **In the evening?**
- **At weekends?**

Every day is different, so note down when the best time for study will be each day. Will there be anyone who can help you with the work if you have problems? Note down times when parents/teachers/workshops/homework or study skills clubs are available. Don't forget that the half or end of term holidays can be a good time to catch up on assignments and revision. Remember to include these in your long–term calculations. However, having completed your planner, will you need to readjust any commitments to give you enough time to complete course work? How important will it be for you to spend some time studying in the day as well as in the evening?

Remember!

Some people can happily juggle an enormous number of different commitments and activities in their lives. They thrive on the variety and the stimulation of so much to do. Others prefer a slower pace, with fewer commitments and more time to concentrate upon each one. How you *find* and *manage* the time you need to complete the course successfully will mean thinking about what conditions *you* need for learning.

Motivation during study periods

It is important to find a place where you can work without interruptions and distractions. Even if you have the luxury of a room and a desk of your own at home, you will probably need to consider using your school, college or public library for some study periods. Settling down to a period of study is easier if you:

- Remove all distractions of hunger, noise, cold and sociable friends!
- Try not to study if you are feeling angry or upset.
- Keep a pad of paper or a jotter next to you as you work. When ideas or other things occur to you, you can note them down before you forget them.
- Give yourself realistic targets and decide for how long you will study before you start. Try not to work for more than an hour without a short break. Reward yourself for completing what you planned to do.
- Try to give yourself a variety of activities to work on.
- Take regular short breaks.
- Have the phone number of someone else from your class or group handy in case you need to check what you need to do or want to discuss the best way to go about a task.

Compiling a portfolio

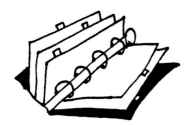

A **portfolio** is a collection of the different types of evidence which can be used to show successful completion of the course. Examples of evidence include:

- Completed **assignments, projects** or **case-studies**, including **action plans** and **evaluations.** These can be in written form or word-processed, although work in the form of **video** recordings, **audio–tape** recordings, **photographs, logbooks** or **diaries** may also be acceptable where they contain evidence of the practical demonstration of skills. Check with your teacher or tutor.

- Past **records of achievement, qualifications, work-experience** or other evidence of 'prior learning'.
- Samples of **relevant class or lecture notes, lists, personal reading records** or **copies of letters** written (perhaps regarding work experience, to request information or advice, or related to job or further education applications).

EQUIPMENT AND MATERIALS

As soon as you know how many compulsory and optional units you will be taking for the course, it will be worthwhile taking advantage of any cheap stationery offers at high street stores and equipping yourself with:

- **At least four large A4 lever arch files** and a set of **extra wide file dividers** (or large **A4 box files**). **One** of these files will become your **portfolio**, the others can be used for organising and storing notes for each compulsory or optional unit and for a "college and course administration" file. (See Figure 5 Filing your material).
- A **hole punch**.
- **File paper**, plain and lined.
- **Plastic pockets or report files**. These are **not** essential but you may feel better if finished assignments are presented neatly in a binder or pocket of some sort. However, do not enclose each individual sheet of an assignment within a plastic pocket. This is expensive, ecologically unsound and drives your teachers and assessors crazy when they have to remove sheets to make comments on your work!
- **Post–it index stickers** can be useful to help 'flag up' important pieces of work, such as evidence for Key Skills certification, in your completed portfolio.
- **Small exercise books or notebooks**, to act as logbooks or diaries.

If you are dyslexic or have another disability which prevents or makes it difficult for you to take notes in lectures, you might consider acquiring a **small tape-recorder** and supply of **tape cassettes**, to enable you to record lectures and play them back at another time.

Reading, note-taking and using a library

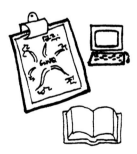

Textbooks such as this can offer you a basic framework for the ideas and information you need for the different subject areas covered in the Intermediate GNVQ in Health and Social Care.

Portfolio

Divide into sections for each:
1. Mandatory unit
2. Optional unit
Use to file completed assignments, projects, case studies or other assessment evidence.
Use post-it index stickers or other labels to show where evidence for Key Skills certification can be found.
Make sure file has a title page and index or contents page.

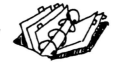

Mandatory units file

This award has 3 Mandatory Units.

Divide your file into sections for each unit.
Use to file class or lecture notes, own notes, articles, references, other relevant information.
It might also be helpful to keep another copy of the Unit descriptions in this file.

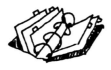

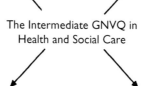

The Intermediate GNVQ in Health and Social Care

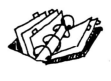

College/school and course administration file

Use this to file:
– Timetable and weekly planners
– Term dates
– Course guides and unit descriptions
– Key Skill requirements
– College or school information
– Library information
– Information from examining board
– Work-experience arrangements

Optional units file

Divide your file into sections for each unit.
Use to file class or lecture notes, own notes, articles, references, other relevant information.
It might also be helpful to keep another copy of the Unit descriptions in this file.

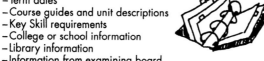

FIGURE 5 *Filing your material.*

Your lectures and classes will supply you with additional material. However, you will need to carry out your own reading and research, making your own notes and updating information in areas where there is constant change (such as social policy legislation, or health advice). It will be useful for you to find out how the national organisation of health and care services works in the area and community in which you live.

You cannot do this successfully without making full use of libraries (including their computers), newspapers and journals, television and film and information produced by a range of national, local and voluntary organisations. If you have personal access to the Internet, you may find such research decidedly easier. Make sure that you are shown how to use all the relevant facilities of your library, whether school, college or public. Use the checklist on page 11 to ensure that you are aware of all the resources on offer.

Using the Internet

Think before reaching for the mouse. Using the Internet can be highly productive but it can take up a lot of your time. Before you start, work out:

● What you need to know.

● How much you need to know.

● When you need the information by.

- Whether you have a sensible search strategy. Do you have list of recommended sites or know how to use an appropriate 'search engine' such as *Yahoo, Lycos* or *Google*?
- Could you find the information you need more easily in books or a journal?

IN MY LIBRARY I CAN:

- Find all shelving where there are books and journals relevant to the subjects covered in this course.   ☐

Make a note of the shelving reference numbers (usually the Dewey System) for health and social care books, sociology, psychology and biology books.   ☐

- use the library's cataloguing and reference facilities, both manual and computerised.   ☐

- operate the photocopying facilities.   ☐

- order books and use any short-term loan arrangement.   ☐

- find and use appropriate reference books such as the British Humanities Index or Social Trends to look up research, articles and statistics relevant to my assignments.   ☐

- access the Internet and download useful material.   ☐

- use CD–ROM facilities for research, e.g. to search through the broad sheet newspapers on disc for relevant articles/information.   ☐

- use the reference section to look up names/addresses and phone numbers of local and national health and social care organisations.   ☐

- find my library membership card!   ☐

Between them, the four sites listed below contain links to literally hundreds of the main health and social care organisations in this country. They are an excellent place from which to start any research.

National Institute for Social work at **www.nisw.org.uk/**

Office for National Statistics at **www.ons.gov.uk/**

King's Fund at **www.kingsfund.org.uk/**

Government Information Service at **www.open.gov.uk**

National Health Service at **www.doh.gov.uk**

Strategies for reading

It is helpful to think of four types of reading: **receptive** and **reflective** reading, **skimming** and **scanning**. All types are useful at some stage in your reading.

Receptive reading is the reading you do most commonly. Reading takes place at a steady easy pace and what is being read is fairly easy to absorb and understand. You may be able to use this type of reading for novels and magazine articles generally related to some of the themes and issues covered in the course.

Reflective reading occurs when you have to think a little more carefully about what you are reading, perhaps because the ideas or information contained in it are new or difficult. You may have to evaluate what you are reading and this may cause you to pause frequently to think about the material.

Skimming through a text, running your eyes down the page fairly rapidly, can give you a good impression of what the material is about and is useful when you need to consider whether or not to spend time reading the material more closely.

Scanning a text also involves running your eyes over a text but in this case you are on the lookout for particular points. It is very useful when looking for answers to particular questions or for specific references.

To be of most use to you, reading will often need to be combined with note-taking.

NOTE-TAKING STRATEGIES

Taking notes *is* time-consuming and requires *active* concentration. Students often worry if:

- they are spending too much time taking endless, detailed notes without really understanding what they will be used for.
- they give up note-taking because they cannot seem to work out what to write down and what not. This can be a particular problem when taking notes in lessons and lectures.

Why take notes? What is note-taking useful for?

Essentially, note-taking is a strategy for helping you **think, understand** and **remember**. There are many situations in life when it is important to focus on the **key issues** or points being communicated. A nurse may have to listen very carefully to a patient describing symptoms of an illness and then later relay this information to other medical staff. A nursery nurse may have to know exactly what to do if a child in her care has an asthma attack or needs adrenaline for a peanut allergy. She may have to explain these things quickly to another person, *summarising essential information*. Both of these health and care workers will have had to have used mental or written note–taking skills, the nurse as she is listening to the patient and the nursery nurse when she first studied the first-aid procedures to apply in emergencies.

Deciding what to write down when you take notes *is* easier if you think about *why* you are taking notes. You may need to take different types of notes for different reasons. You will get better at working out methods of note–taking which suit you the more you try out different approaches. It also helps to think about ways to *store* your notes so that they are easily accessible to you when you need them. If they are written or designed in such a way that you can make use of them again, you will be more likely to come back to them.

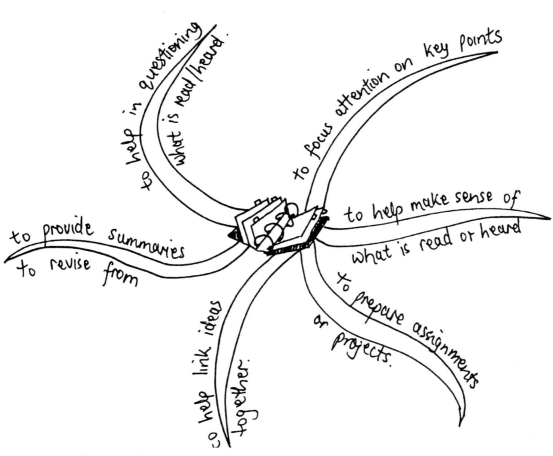

FIGURE 6 *Different uses for notes.*

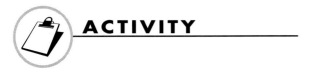 **ACTIVITY**

Three different methods for taking notes are summarised below. Working individually or as a small group, *experiment* with these methods for:

- **taking notes from this textbook**
- **taking notes from a lecture**
- **taking notes from a relevant television documentary**

Discuss and compare the results of your experiments with each method. Which method did you feel most comfortable with? Did you find yourself writing too little or too much? How much time did the exercise take? Would you find the notes useful to read again? What would you use the notes for?

Three methods for taking notes:

- Mind-mapping
- Underlining and Highlighting
- PQ4R

1 Mind-Mapping

Visual thinkers may find this technique, described on page 20, extremely useful for summarising keypoints and issues.

2 Underlining and highlighting

If you own the book or article you are taking notes from, highlighting, underlining and marking the margin with asterisks or other symbols can be a quick and effective method of skim–reading a text, focusing your attention on it and getting to grips with the material as a whole.

3 PQ4R

Linear and sequential thinkers (those who like to plot the logical connections between items of information or arguments) may find the note–taking method known as PQ4R worth adopting.

Preview

Question

Read

Reflect

Recite

Review

Preview

Before you begin to read your chapter, article or book:

- Stop! Look at the title, the contents page and the date the book was published.
- Read any introduction.
- Scan the section you are reading for headings, subheadings and key passages.
- Look at the pictures, charts, graphs and other visual images.

All these activities will help you gain an impression of the main points and key issues covered in the text.

Question

Now ask yourself:

- What am I likely to learn from this text?
- Is this material from which I need to extract a *lot* or a *little* information? How useful will the information be to me?
- What questions is the author asking?

Read

Read carefully through the material, rereading difficult passages. Stop and think about what you have read.

Reflect

Make notes on the key issues, information or ideas in the text. As you do so, **question** what you note down. Do you *agree* with what you are reading? Do you think the author has missed important points, evidence or issues? Which points/information seem particularly important or crucial? Are there terms, names or dates which you think you may need to remember or come back to? Is there any information or ideas which would help you to write an assignment? Has something the author has written helped you understand another issue?

Recite

If the text you are taking notes on contains information you need to memorise (perhaps for a test) without looking at the text, recite to yourself quietly or out loud the main points. Reread the text or your notes if you cannot do this.

Review

Check, when trying to recall the main points of this text, your notes make sense. You may need to make a shorter summary of your longer notes. Use coloured pens and symbols, jot down key words and phrases and ideas, diagrams or sketches onto a smaller card(using a card index file can help). Now try to convert these shortened notes into your own words, either orally or in writing.

It is sometimes said that we now live in a world of **information overload**. The growth of the mass media and in particular the Internet means that we are bombarded daily with information, ideas and viewpoints from a huge number of sources. The ability to extract what is useful and discard what is not from what you read, see and hear is essential to avoid overload and confusion. Note-taking can help you acquire this skill.

Writing assignments, projects and case-studies

Why assess through course work?

Two-thirds of the Intermediate GNVQ in Health and Social Care is assessed through course work. Most of this course work is set in the form of assignments, projects or case–studies. Why is your work being assessed in this way, rather than, for instance, through examinations? There are five main reasons:

● to allow you to *make your own contribution to* — put your own stamp on — each subject or topic–related assignment.

● to support you while encouraging you to *use your own initiative* in solving problems, answering questions and completing tasks set.

● to enable you to see each assignment you do to *acquire a deeper knowledge and understanding* of the area you are studying **and** to *reflect critically on the ways in which you learn.*

● to provide opportunities to *work with others* and *gain confidence* in approaching your teachers, tutors, lecturers, friends, and others working in health and social care organisations for help, extra information, the exchange of views, work experience and the acquisition of practical skills.

● to, ultimately, *put you in charge of your own learning.* To enable you to work out, after you have finished a piece of work, what you have learnt and what you still need to know, what was easy and what was more difficult and how you would improve it given another chance. To give you the ability to know when your work is good or good enough without over–relying on the approval and assessments of others. Finally, to allow you to transfer the appropriate skills and knowledge to any future study or work. When you can do this you will have well-developed *meta-cognitive skills,* i.e. you can "think about thinking" and reflect upon your own learning style and strategies, choosing those most appropriate to a task.

Working out what an assignment requires you to do needs to be approached actively and positively.

Ask yourself these questions:

1 Why am I doing this?
2 What do I have to do here?
3 What will be the best way to approach this task?
4 Do I need to change the way I am tackling this piece of work?
5 How can I improve what I am doing?
6 Have I other skills I could use to help me with this task?

Sometimes assignments can be written in ways which make it difficult to work out what to do and how to begin.

Look at these three typical assignment tasks:

- **Analyse** the different ways in which people cope with change and how these changes could affect the type of help and support they need.
- **Analyse** the effectiveness of codes of practice and charters in upholding the care value base.
- **Evaluate** your communication strategies accurately, identifying strengths and ways to improve on weaknesses.

When reading assignment titles, if you are unsure what is meant by words such as **analyse and evaluate**, use the *Key Words and Phrases Table* on page 18 to help you work out what assignments involve. **Brainstorm** the wording of the task, trying to note down anything you think might be relevant.

Example

Task: Analyse the effectiveness of codes of practice and charters in upholding the care value base.

The result of a brainstorm exercise on this task might look like this:

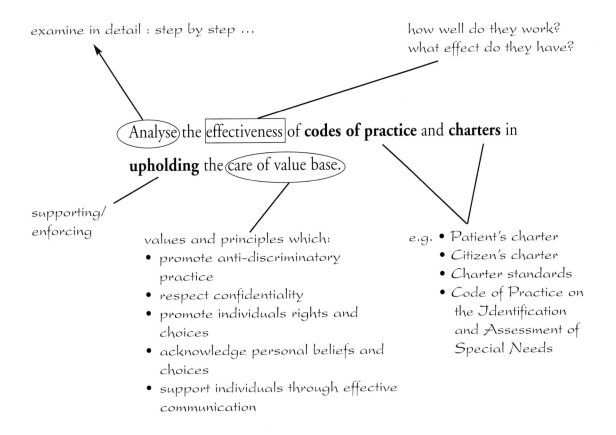

FIGURE 7 *Decoding assignment tasks.*

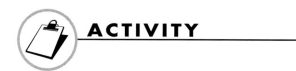

ACTIVITY

Now carry out a similar exercise for the other assignment tasks identified on page 17 (or others you have been given at your school/college). If you are working in a group or a class, compare and discuss your interpretations of the questions.

● **Analyse**   examine in detail: separate into component parts

If we analyse our survey into teenage smoking, we find that girls generally start smoking at an earlier age to boys.

● **Compare**   look for differences and similarities.

A comparison of the Sex Discrimination and Race Relations Act shows that they both make a distinction between indirect and direct discrimination.

● **Critically evaluate**   use evidence to support your judgements.

Mary's critical evaluation of child poverty in Britain discussed evidence from large and small-scale research studies.

● **Describe**   give a written, visual or oral account, as required

I described the Greentrees Home for the Elderly as well-resourced, warm and welcoming, sympathetic to the needs of its occupants and forward thinking.

● **Explain**   make clear and give reasons for: help others understand.

Most teenagers would benefit from an exact explanation of the effects of oestrogen and progesterone on the body during puberty:

● **Identify**   pick out key characteristics. What is most important?

Ishmael identified the key characteristics of a good piece of research as readability, validity and relevance.

● **Discuss**   consider an issue from various points of view.

In my report I discussed different views on the use of "politically correct" language in health and care work.

TABLE 2 *Assignments – Key Words and Phrases.*

ORGANISING IDEAS AND ACTION PLANNING

When you have worked out what the assignment requires you to do, you need to consider:

- How to collect together the information you need. Where will you find suitable information or source material? Who can help you or give you the information you need? What range of sources will you be expected to use?
- How to consult other people (teachers, friends, tutors), who can give you ideas for completing the work. During formal discussions (class or tutorial) you could consider using a Dictaphone or a tape-recorder to record useful ideas that are given.
- How, if you are working as a group, you will hold meetings and share out the tasks.

Techniques for organising and generating ideas

Brainstorm techniques, spider diagrams and mind–maps are all worth exploring as methods for coming up with ideas for each task in the assignment and then linking them together.

Brainstorming is particularly useful if you are working in a group. Alone, or with others, simply note down any useful ideas, words, visual images, arguments or information relevant to the question being discussed. **Spider diagrams** are helpful if you haven't much time and need a rough sketch of what a piece of work will involve. They can help you begin to structure and link material and ideas together.

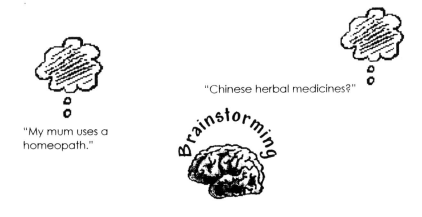

How many areas of complementary medicine exist?

"My mum uses a homeopath."

"Chinese herbal medicines?"

"Osteopaths can help with back pain, I think."

"Is reflexology where feet are massaged?"

FIGURE 8 *Using brainstorming techniques to generate ideas.*

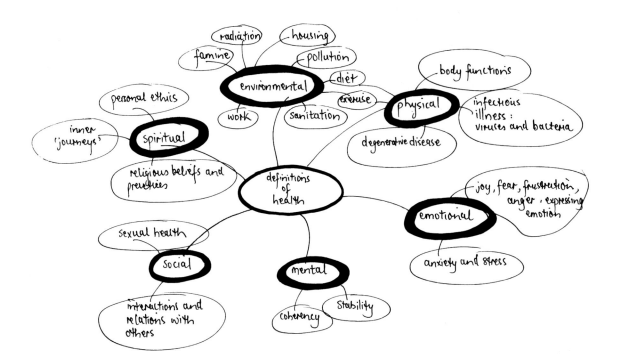

FIGURE 9 *Use spider diagrams.*

MIND-MAPPING

This is a very useful technique for *visual learners* who find it easier to organise their thoughts and ideas in linked key words and pictures This method can be used for generating ideas and planning your work as well as, later on, note–taking and revising.

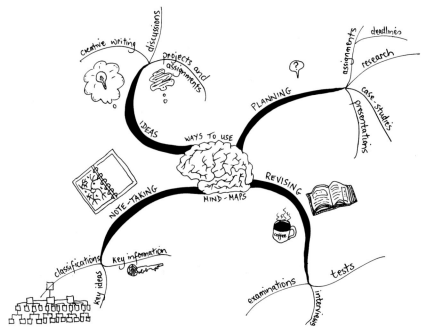

FIGURE 10 *Ways to use mind-mapping.*

USING MIND-MAPPING

- In the centre of your page draw a picture, or name in words, your main topic or theme.
- draw branches from this main topic in thick lines (use different colours or patterns). Label your branches with key words and/or images.
- Draw sub–branches from the main branches to represent sub–topics or to elaborate and extend your ideas. Again, use key words, phrases, images, pictures and colour. Use italics, underlining and capitals to highlight your work.

Let your ideas flow and develop. Add more details to your mind–map as ideas occur to you. However, the mind–map is not meant to be an art–form, more a way to focus your attention on the essential components of a piece of work, topic or report.

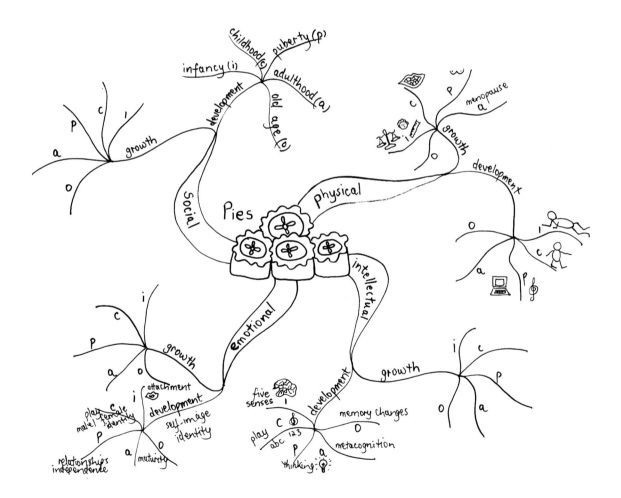

FIGURE 11 *A mind–map in progress: 'Factors to consider in human growth and development'.*

Planning and prioritising tasks

If you use a planner regularly it is easier to break up assignments and projects into a series of smaller tasks, each of which you could aim to complete within a manageable time such as an hour or two. Subdividing your course work in this way also allows you to **prioritise** the tasks. In what order are they best done? Which really need to be done straightaway? Make a list of small tasks in order of priority with the time you estimate they will take and target dates for completion. Leave room on your action plan to amend these dates when and if your plan is modified.

Example: Breaking down an assignment into smaller tasks.

Nadia has been asked to complete the following assignment.

Produce a report on human development based on one or more case studies. It must include:

- characteristics of the different life stages

- factors which have affected personal development and self–concept

- changes which have happened in a person's life

- examples of support used by an individual in the case–study or studies

This is her Action-Plan

Action plan

- Phone aunt Santha. Can I use my cousin Paul (12 years old) for one of my case–studies?

  Arrange to interview aunt Santha and Paul. Time **10 mins.** Complete by: **2nd October**

- Phone my mum's friend Sundner, who is getting married next month, to ask if I can interview him for the second case-study. Arrange a time to see him.

  Time: **10 mins.** Complete by: **2nd October**

- Prepare my interview schedule for both case–studies. Use my class notes and textbook for ideas about the questions to include. Type up interview schedules. Ask tutor to check them for me.

  Time: **2 hours.** Complete by: **4th October**

- Make sure I have film for my camera so I can take photos of Paul and Sunder for my assignments. Has aunt Santha any photos of Paul growing up that she can spare?

  Time: **10 mins** Complete by: **5th October**

- Make notes on the main theories of development which relate to my case–studies.

  Time: **1 hour** Complete by: **8th October**

- Carry out out interviews. Type up case–studies on computer, relating the results of my interviews to the theories.

  Time: **3 hours** Complete by: **12th October**

- Redraft whole assignment, using spell-checker on computer to correct errors.

  Time: **15 mins**. Complete by: **14th October**

- **Total time I need** Approx **7 hours** : Plot out when I can fit this in on weekly planners. Check date assignment has to be given in: **16 October**

Monitoring and revising your work

There are likely to be many points during the completion of a piece of course work when you will change direction or modify your original plan in some way. **On your action plan, keep a note of:**

- the reasons for changing your plans
- what new plans you have for the work

 ## ACTIVITY

Use the example of Nadia's action plan to help you prepare an action plan for your first set assignment. You may find that your school or college will give you an action–planning form to fill in for each assignment. If not, it will be quite acceptable for you to invent your own along the lines of the example above. Use your IT skills to prepare a format which you could use to save time on each new piece of work.

....

Writing skills

Introducing new material, connecting points and paragraphs, writing conclusions

When you have reached the point when you want to start writing the assignment, you need to think about the quality of the language you are going to use to convey your ideas. Problems can crop up when...

- you are unsure whether the assignment should be written in an academic, formal style (*"it can be argued that. . ."*) or whether it is acceptable to use the first–person (*"I found that..."*). Check with the person who set the assignment.

- you have difficulty with the **flow** of the writing, especially when critically evaluating or analysing an issue from several different perspectives or when there is a lot of conflicting evidence. Use the **"Linking words and phrases"** checklist on page 24 to help you write an introduction and link each paragraph to the next one, introducing new ideas and points in a clear way without losing sight of the original aims of the report.

- you reach the end of the report and need to draw ideas together and write an evaluation and/or conclusion. You need to avoid abrupt, over–brief evaluations. Instead use "**A guide to GNVQ evaluation**" on page 25 to help you show that you have reflected and analysed the issues involved as well as considered your own "performance".

● you are aware that there are significant weaknesses in spelling, punctuation or grammar in your work. If you use a word–processor make sure that you know how to use a spell–checker and then use this as a matter of routine whenever you finish a piece of work. If you are dyslexic and standard spell–checking programmes do not pick up all your errors, there are some useful software applications. Some of these are expensive but check if you are entitled to recoup some or all of the costs under the Disabled Students Allowance Scheme (see page 53).

INTRODUCTORY PARAGRAPHS

In this report/assignment/case-study I intend to…
This report will discuss/analyse/examine/compare/evaluate…
There are two/three/four theories which need to be considered…
There are several areas of this debate…

CONNECTING EACH POINT AND/OR PARAGRAPH

It can be argued that…
Some writers suggest that…
Nevertheless…
On the other hand…
At first sight…
'X; argues that… whereas "y" suggests that…
Caution needs to be exercised in interpreting these results because…
In her discussion/analysis of…
Arguably…
What is interesting about this view is…
This theory implies that…
As we have seen…

CONCLUDING REMARKS

In conclusion…
This evidence/research confirms that…
There is insufficient evidence in this research to…
While this policy has benefited…, it has been of less value to…

To summarise:
In short…
What this idea fails to recognise is…

TABLE 3 *Checklist: Linking words and phrases.*

Evaluating a piece of work is not necessarily exactly the same as *concluding* it. When writing a conclusion to an assignment, the key issues or experiences discussed in the work can be fully summarised and, depending on the kind of assignment or project, judgements may be made about the validity or reliability of the theories or evidence discussed. The ideas and knowledge covered by the course can be complex. Good conclusions should reflect the fact that different points of view exist and different solutions to problems need to be assessed.

However, **GNVQ evaluation** offers you the opportunity to review retrospectively your entire approach to completing the assignment. You may be asked to consider whether the way in which you tackled the work was appropriate. Can you justify the approach you took to the work? Could you have done the work differently? What could you have done to improve the work? You are being encouraged to look critically at your own learning and performance on the course. It is important to realise that you are **not** expected to produce perfect work from the very beginning of your studies. However, if you take the time to evaluate your work carefully, you will soon become much more aware of the ways in which your knowledge, skills and understanding can improve.

When evaluating a course work assignment, you should...

● Check the original requirements of the assignment. Have you met them all? Show the ways in which you could have done so.

● What approaches to the assignment did you consider and actually use? Which worked well and which did not? Why?

● What skills does your assignment demonstrate?

● What improvements would you make if you did this piece of work again and why?

TABLE 4 *A guide to GNVQ evaluation.*

All students with spelling or word-finding difficulties could consider the use of a **hand-held electronic spell-checker**. These are relatively inexpensive (£12.00 – £30.00) and some models also include a thesaurus (i.e. a list of words with similar meanings), a calculator, games, grammar guides etc.). Franklin make some of the best models which are easily available from high–street stores such as Argos.

Proof-reading and editing your work.

At this level of study, it is **not** acceptable to hand in first drafts of work. Presentation is important (just as it would be if you were preparing a report in the workplace) so you will be expected to check your own errors. Some of the resources mentioned above may help you but as a general rule, the use of a dictionary, spell–checker and thesaurus should become automatic. If you are uncertain about how to check your own work, consider the advice below on proof-reading.

PROOF-READING

When you read over something you have written, to look for mistakes, it is called proof-reading.

You can look for different kinds of mistakes, like:

- **Missing capital letters**
- **Capitals where there shouldn't be capitals**
- **Missing full stops, commas or other kinds of punctuation**
- **Sentences that don't make sense**
- **Spelling mistakes**

Proof-reading can be easier if…

- You **leave some time** between doing the writing and proofreading it: it makes it easier to spot the mistakes.
- You proof-read for **one kind of mistake at a time.** You may miss a lot if you try to correct everything at once.
- You try, when proof-reading for spelling mistakes, **starting with the last word and then checking the second last word and so on**. This makes spelling mistakes jump out at you much more.
- You decide **how much** proof-reading you really need to do. Some pieces of work, like assignments, projects and case-studies, do need very careful proof-reading. Other work, like a note you have written for yourself, just needs checking that it makes sense.

Presentation skills

How much care do you take over the presentation of your work? Use Table 5 to work out your own strengths and weaknesses in this respect. Students on this course will also be actively encouraged to develop their skills in the use of information technology. One way in which you can vastly improve the presentation of your work is by typing or word-processing all or part of it. If you can touch type this will be much easier. There are several good touch-typing programmes available for anyone with access to a computer and CD ROM drive. These are listed in the Resources section at the end of this chapter.

PRESENTATION SKILLS

When I look through my work I notice that: (Tick any which apply to you)

1 I usually put the **date** of the work. ☐

2 I usually make sure my work has a **title** and it is **underlined**. ☐

3 My writing is **legible** or I **type** my work. Other people can easily read what I have written. ☐

4 I **do not** leave **large gaps or spaces** between sections of my writing. ☐

5 If I need to number my work, the **numbering is clear**. ☐

6 I draw **clear diagrams** and **tables**. ☐

7 I always **label** my diagrams and tables neatly, using a ruler where necessary. ☐

8 I use plenty of **colour** in my pictures and illustrations. ☐

9 **Loose worksheets** are **attached carefully** to my books or files. ☐

10 **I finish off any work at home** which I did not have time to finish in class. ☐

11 I try to **correct my own work**, proof-reading or redrafting pieces of work before I hand them in to be marked. ☐

12 **I correct my own spelling mistakes**, using a spell checker, or ask someone to help me. ☐

13 **Good presentation of my work** seems to help me achieve better grades. ☐

TABLE 5 *Presentation Skills.*

Writing a bibliography

You will be expected to write a bibliography (a list of books, articles, and other resources used) for each assignment you submit. To do this properly, you need to make a note of your materials and references as you study. There is nothing worse than finishing an assignment and then spending valuable time hunting down the name of a book you read in the library but did not note the details of. As a general rule, you need to note:

● the title of the book or article (or web site address)
● the author(s)
● the publisher
● the date of publication
● the place of publication

Examples

Book:

Thomson, H. Holden C. Aslangul S, (2000) *Intermediate GNVQ Health and Social Care,* London, Hodder and Stoughton.

Article:

Benn, M. (1999), 'The politics of poverty', *Community Care Magazine,* 9–15 September 1999.

Reader:

(i.e. a book containing many articles or chapters by different authors).

Domielli, L (1992) "An uncaring profession? An examination of racism in social work', *Racism and Antiracism — Inequalities, Opportunities and Policies.* Eds: P. Braham, A. Rutanski, R. Skellington. London: Sage.

Other sources of information or references in your work may come from the **Internet** (give the web site address), **workplace** (acknowledge the source), **television programmes, video or film** (give the title and date) or **friends, family and teachers** (attribute information as accurately as you can).

Meeting grading requirements

Work for the Intermediate Level GNVQ in Health and Social Care will be graded at one of three grades, Pass, Merit or Distinction. Each complete unit will receive a grade, worth a number of points, which will then be added together to give a grade for the whole qualification. The Unit Descriptions for the course contain a detailed account of the type of work necessary to achieve grades at Pass, Merit or Distinction. In addition, each Unit Description includes examples of ways in which students can develop evidence for the three Key Skills of *communication, application of number* and *information technology.* Make sure you are given as copy of the Unit Descriptions for your file.

Memory skills and techniques: the importance of review

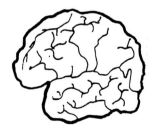

One of the compulsory units of the Intermediate GNVQ Health and Social Care is externally assessed. One method of external assessment *may* be tests. The Key Skills Qualification will also be assessed through a mixture of internal and external assessments, including some tests.

There may also be occasions during your course when your teachers feel it is important to ask you to memorise material.

However, compared to students taking, for example, GCSE courses, students taking this GNVQ will have less information and fewer ideas and arguments to memorise. They will not be expected to write essays or extended answers to questions under test conditions.

WHAT DO TIMED TESTS ASSESS?

Consider this situation

Sharmeena is a nursery nurse at a day nursery for under fives. Parents normally pick up the children at 5.30 p.m. On Friday, Paul, Josie's father, turns up fifteen minutes early, clearly drunk and demanding to take his daughter home immediately. Paul does not live with Josie's mother and there is an agreement that he picks up Josie on Mondays and Tuesdays, and Pat, Josie's mother, picks her up on the other three weekdays.

Sharmeena has answered the door to Paul, who is now shouting at her in the reception area of the nursery building. He is swearing and threatening to push Sharmeena out of the way if she does not let him into the room where the children are playing.

Though feeling nervous, Sharmeena has fortunately **remembered three key pieces** of advice given her at a training course on facing aggression in the workplace:

- stay calm and use positive, not negative, words and phrases to help change the emotion of the aggressor.
- offer to reward good behaviour.
- firmly and gently explain how the aggressor's behaviour is affecting you.

Sharmeena suggests to Paul that she can help him if he stops shouting. She says that she will talk to her supervisor to see what she can do to help, adding that his shouting is making her feel nervous although she is sure that a solution to the problem could be found. Although still tense and red–faced, Paul calms down enough to listen to the nursery manager, who has now arrived at the scene. He agrees to wait to talk to Josie's mother and, in the intervening ten minutes, reveals that there have been problems between Pat and himself over access to Josie.

There are many situations like this in working life where, under pressure, it will have been important or even crucial (for example, where first–aid knowledge has had to be applied) to have memorised key information or ideas.

In more routine working situations, it will, of course, be possible if necessary, to check one's understanding or memory by consulting reference manuals, books or colleagues. The ability to use a skill will also become more automatic with practice. Nevertheless, being required to memorise something is good rehearsal for real–life pressures and crises. GNVQ tests are therefore designed to give you practice in:

- reviewing key information, ideas and theories.
- developing and understanding effective memory techniques.
- writing short responses to stimulus questions under timed test conditions.

Preparing for tests

1 Overcoming examination nerves

We feel nervous when we do not feel confident. Tests and examinations may make us feel nervous for very good reasons. We are under pressure to show what we can do or what we know. Our 'performance' may be measured against the performance of other people around us. It would be strange, therefore, if we did not feel anxious!

Some anxiety is natural and may actually help us in tests and examinations. If we are 'keyed–up' for a test, we are concentrating hard and focusing on what we have to do. We **want** to succeed. If we could not care less and are totally relaxed, we may not have enough adrenaline speeding through our system to keep us going throughout the test.

Too much anxiety and nerves can also be a problem. It can make our minds 'go blank' just when we need to remember what we have learnt or concentrate on a problem. Some people feel most anxious about performance tests such as a driving test or a piano examination. Other people worry more about written tests. A person may be good at remembering facts but less confident about puzzling out which of several likely answers in a multiple choice question is the best one to choose.

2 Ensuring adequate preparation: the importance of review

One of the surest ways of avoiding too much panic is to allow yourself the time and energy to prepare carefully for the tests:

- make sure you know which of your course units will be externally tested and when the tests will take place. Will you be given another chance to take the tests if you do not do as well as you hoped the first time round?
- gather all the information and advice you can find on what you need to learn for the test by consulting your course guide, your class notes, your textbooks, teachers and peers. Ask to see some practice test papers.
- Start the process of revision and review well in advance of the test date, using your weekly planner to assign short but regular 'chunks' of time to test preparation. Figure 12 'The importance of review', demonstrates how effective such regular boosts to your memory can be.

THE IMPORTANCE OF REVIEWING

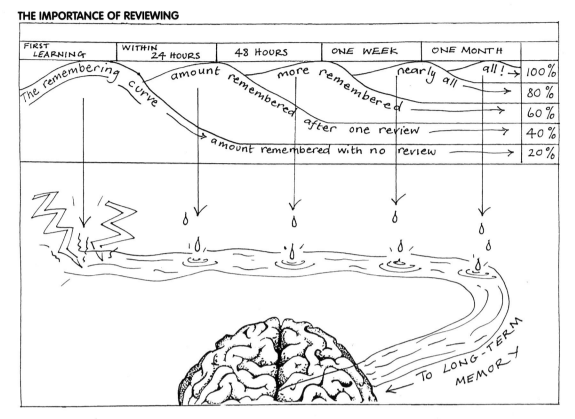

FIGURE 12 *The importance of reviewing.*

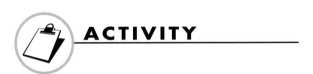 **ACTIVITY**

Try out the theory demonstrated in Figure 12 yourself. Over a period of a month, choose a particular section of information which you need to learn for a test. Plot out on your weekly planner or diary fifteen minutes revision of this material within 24 hours, 28 hours, one week and a month of first trying to learn it. Try to keep to this revision plan and at the end, assess whether the material has been learned effectively.

(Alternatively, persuade a teacher or lecturer to build in this experimental exercise into their class time).

3 Understanding memory

Explore different methods for remembering your material (see Figure 13 – Make your memory work). Information can be remembered in many ways and finding strategies which work for you will give you an insight into how your memory works and how you can use it more effectively.

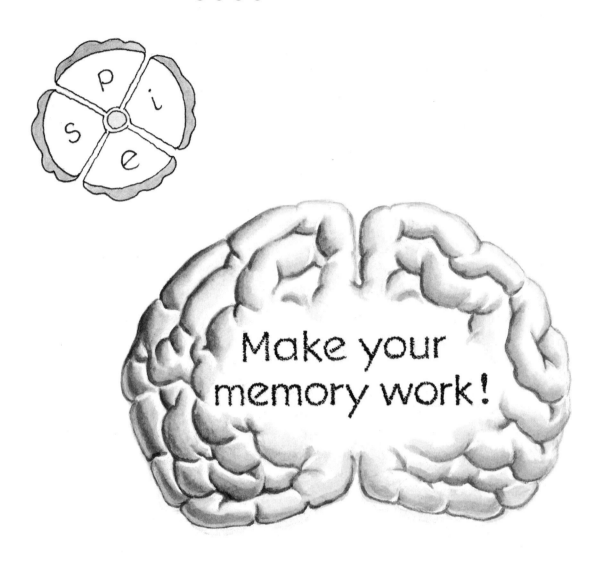

Make your
memory work!

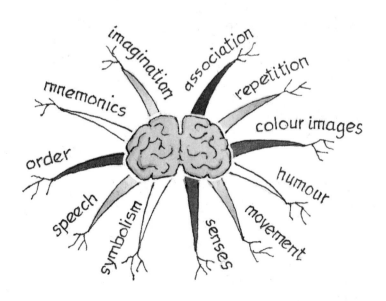

FIGURE 13 *Make your memory work.*

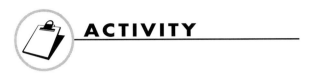

ACTIVITY

Look at Table 6, *'Legislation and organisations which challenge discrimination,'* for five minutes. Try to remember as much as you can without writing anything down. Now cover the table and try to write down everything you remember.

In groups or individually, discuss and consider:

- the strategies you used to remember the contents of the table. Did these include any of the strategies described in Figure 13?
- what additional strategies (written, verbal, other) might have been effective?
- what would you need to do to retain this information for a test in a month's time?

....

Sex Discrimination Act 1975	The Commission for Racial Equality	Disability Discrimination Act 1995
The European Court of Justice	The Equal Opportunities Commission	The European Convention on Human Rights
Race Relations Act 1976	The Disability Rights Commission	Fair Employment Act (Northern Ireland) 1989

TABLE 6 *Legislation and organisations which challenge discrimination.*

TEST TECHNIQUES

When the day of a test arrives, give yourself plenty of time to check everything; check equipment, have breakfast, arrive on time but not too early. Try not to talk about the test with friends before you start. Have a last look at any brief notes or summaries you have made. As soon as you are allowed to, read the questions. Make sure you understand the test instructions. Ask for help if necessary. **Take your time**. Highlight keywords and note down any key facts you know you will have to use at some point but may forget as the test proceeds. If you suffer from acute 'nerves', give yourself something to smile about and imagine (just briefly!) the teachers in charge of the examinations in a nudist camp. If all else fails, take a few deep breaths and tell yourself that you are not going to let the test get the better of you. Start with the questions you feel most confident with first and then tackle the rest.

Answer all the questions. Time and pace yourself. Keep an eye on the clock or a watch. Be strict about keeping within the time–limits for the questions. If you have time left at the end of the test, proof–read and check your answers.

Keep tests in perspective. It will be great if you do well because you will enjoy feeling successful but if you do not, it is not the end of the world. You can always do things differently next time.

Special assessment concessions

The teachers of students with certain disabilities, illnesses or exceptional circumstances (including dyslexic and dyspraxic students) can, on their behalf, make a request to the examining board for special test arrangements (such as extra time) and/or special consideration (action taken after the examination). If you think you are eligible for, and could benefit from these concessions, discuss this with your teacher and tutors as far in advance of the tests as possible, preferably at the beginning of your course.

Giving Oral Presentations

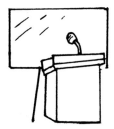

Lena has coped with assignments, tests and work–experience but then she is asked to give a short oral presentation to her class on the research project she has been carrying out. Her friend Adam said that when he did his talk he quite enjoyed the change to speak uninterrupted for a full ten minutes but Lena would rather be forced to commit the entire NHS and Community Care Act to memory than stand up and speak in front of an audience, even one she knows as well as her GNVQ group.

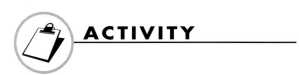

ACTIVITY

1 Are you a 'Lena' or an 'Adam' (or perhaps something in between)? What advice would you offer to both Lena and Adam to ensure that Lena can overcome her nervousness and Adam can avoid giving a rambling or boring talk?

2 You may well be given the opportunity to give a short talk or presentation to enable you to develop greater self-confidence and to acquire a skill which is often used in working in health and care occupations. For example, a ward manager in a hospital may have to brief doctors and paramedics about the condition of patients in her care or a social worker may have to talk to groups of prospective foster parents. Can you think of any other situations where health and social care workers may need to address groups of colleagues, clients, patients, service–users or the general public?

Preparation

● Think about the **purpose** of the presentation. In what ways should your audience benefit from the talk? Are you hoping to give them information or do you hope to discuss ideas and theories? Do you want your audience to participate in your presentation in anyway or is the purpose of the talk to give a briefing? How will you keep your listeners interested in what you say? Will you use handouts or audio–visual aids, such as slides or an overhead projector? Will you use tape–recordings, music, clips from video or television programmes? If so, you will need to ensure that the equipment is ready and set up for you to use.

- Consider the length of the presentation and practice what you want to say in that time. Try not to overrun your allotted time.

- Try not to read out from a script. Instead, make notes of the key points you want to make on cue–cards and practise using these to put together your talk. A punchy and interesting introduction and conclusion to the talk always helps.

- Make sure you research and prepare your material carefully and stick to the "brief" you are given for the talk.

- If you feel very nervous about giving a presentation alone, ask if you could 'pair up' with a fellow student to give a joint talk.

DELIVERY

- It can be very helpful to use "cueing words" throughout your talk to help it flow along. You will probably use some of these automatically but a quick glance at Table 7 may help you choose some other useful phrases.

- Consider your posture and movements as you talk. Will you stand or sit, stay in one place or move around the room?

- Try to speak clearly and avoid fixing our gaze on one or two people, especially your friends! Try to make everyone in the room feel included in your presentation.

---

1 SEQUENCE SIGNALS (*I'M PUTTING MY IDEAS IN AN ORDER.*)

first, second, third	in the first place, second place etc.
then	next
before	now
after	while
until	last(ly)
during	since
always	later / earlier

---

2 ILLUSTRATION SIGNALS (*THIS IS WHAT I MEAN*)

for example	specifically
for instance	to illustrate
such as	much like
in the same way as	similar to

3 CONTINUATION SIGNALS (*I'VE MORE IDEAS TO COME*)

and	also	another
again	and finally	first of all
a final reason	furthermore	in addition
last of all	likewise	more
moreover	next	one reason
other	secondly	similarly
too	with	

4 CHANGE OF DIRECTION SIGNALS (*WATCH OUT – I'M GOING BACK OVER SOMETHING*)

although	but	conversely
despite	different from	even though
however	in contrast	instead of
in spite of	nevertheless	otherwise
the opposite	on the contrary	on the other hand
rather	still	yet
while	though	

5 EMPHASIS SIGNALS (*I'M SAYING SOMETHING IMPORTANT NOW*)

a major development	it all boils down to
a significant factor	most of all
a key feature	more than anything else
remember that	it should be noted
above all	especially important
especially relevant	important to note

TABLE 7

CONFIDENCE AND SELF-ESTEEM

Even if, like Lena in the story above, you are nervous **before** the talk, **after** it is over you should feel a great sense of achievement. With luck you should not find it so difficult to contemplate doing another presentation. There are many techniques for handling 'nerves', including taking deep breaths before you start but often the first few words are the worst. Once you have begun speaking and are concentrating on your material, feelings of nervousness often recede or disappear and you find that you can complete the talk. There will be plenty of people in your group who feel exactly the same as you do about giving talks and their sympathies will be with you!

Make sure that you are given the opportunity to discuss how the presentation went with a teacher or tutor. Your fellow students will also give you plenty of informal 'feedback' but it is sometimes helpful if they are encouraged to offer comments within the classroom.

Working collaboratively

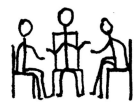

Television dramas such as *Casualty* and *E.R* have provided us with vivid images of how positive, successful and sometimes essential it can be for health and care workers to work collaboratively, offering different skills and expertise and contributing ideas based on varied experiences and training. Most health and social care workers, whatever their individual roles and responsibilities, work as part of a wider 'team'. Problems which affect staff and service users, patients or clients are discussed in meetings or supervision sessions and the improvement of the service as a whole becomes a shared responsibility.

However, it would not be true to claim that, within all health and social care services, team or group work always operates effectively. Much depends on the structure of the organisation, the size of and hierarchies within departments, the type and quality of management and on group dynamics, i.e. how individuals within working groups or teams interact professionally and personally.

Some of the factors may affect the success of group work assignments you may be asked to participate in. If your class or group has been encouraged, from the start of the course, to get to know each other well, to discuss issues in a non-threatening atmosphere of mutual respect and there have been many opportunities for whole or small-group work, a group assignment will be more likely to be a productive and positive experience. It will also be an opportunity to develop and record evidence for your portfolio of competence in the key skills of problem-solving and working with others. The tables on page 38 should help you to plan group work projects, assessing your own skills and avoiding some of the pitfalls.

1 Allow problems in the group or team itself to be aired and discussed.

2 Make sure everyone in the team knows what the team has to do, has taken part in planning the work and understands their role.

3 Talk to each other!

4 Value everyone's contribution and role and encourage and praise each other's work.

5 If appropriate, give someone in the group a co-ordinating role.

6 Try not to allow groups or teams to become too big or too small.

7 Give yourself time to 'gel' as a group.

8 Make sure you have somewhere to work – a base – and, if necessary, somewhere to keep materials, equipment etc.

9 Discuss how you will make decisions and make them jointly. Be prepared to change or review your procedures.

10 Review regularly how the team is working and what progress it is making.

TABLE 8 *How to work well in teams.*

The following statements reflect a wide range of possible roles. Which of these group roles do you generally take on?

ROLE	MOST OF THE TIME	SOME OF THE TIME	NEVER
Acting as peacemaker, trying to smooth problems and reduce tensions in the group			
Acting as the group clown or joker			
Being creative and original with ideas and views			
Being picked on or bullied by other group members			
Caring and looking after other group members who might be upset or uncomfortable			
Challenging and confronting views of behaviour of which you disapprove			
Constantly drawing others back to the task if they wander			
Constantly drawing the group back to its task or agenda			
Disrupting or sabotaging the formal agenda in order to follow your own			

Drawing out possible hidden agendas or feelings that may be blocking progress	
Encouraging and motivating others to contribute	
Encouraging others to be creative and original	
Initiating discussion or activities	
Keeping others focused on group task and purpose	
Listening quietly until you can see an opening to contribute	
Unhelpful stirring or winding other people up	

TABLE 9 *Contributing to a Group.*

SUMMARY PERSONAL FEELINGS ABOUT GROUP PARTICIPATION	YOUR ASSESSMENT	OTHERS' ASSESSMENT, E.G. TEACHER/LECTURER/PEERS/ WORK-EXPERIENCE SUPERVISOR
Are you reasonably comfortable when taking part in a group activity or discussion? What reasons would you give for your answer?		
What do you think that you contribute to a group i.e. consider your strong points?		
What difficulties or problems do you meet when in a group?		
Are you confident of being able to lead or manage a group or group activity?		
Have you the skills to lead or manage a group or group activity?		

When contributing to, leading or managing a group do you always plan and prepare well? How important do you think it is to be well prepared?
What kind of leadership do you provide?
How effective is it?
How might you improve your leadership skills?
How do you think you could improve your contributions to a group and group work skills

Permission to reproduce this document is given by Stonham Housing Association Ltd

DISCUSSION

Well-managed class discussions can bring your course to life. Listening to and responding to other peoples' ideas can help you to think through your own beliefs and opinions. Strong differences of opinion or perspective within a group can spark heated debate. A quieter, thoughtful exchange of ideas can help you appreciate an issue or subject more clearly. Some people have few inhibitions about participating in discussions, but if discussions are dominated by just a few students they can become unsatisfactory and less enjoyable for the whole group.

If you find it difficult to join in discussions, try the following strategies:

- **Listen to** a specific point the teacher or another student has made. **Ask a question, make a comment** about it or **offer an example or illustration** of it as early in the discussion as possible. When you have made a contribution, feelings of nervousness may recede and you may find it easier to contribute again.
- **Help others reluctant to contribute** by asking them questions, appealing to experience or views you know they have. Try to share in the responsibility for keeping the discussion alive.
- **Help the group to stay focused on the subject** or purpose of the discussion, especially if there is a task to complete afterwards. If the discussion seems to be straying from the point, offer a contribution such as "*shall we go back to the question of...*" or "*so let's recap...*".

Discussions can also fall flat if only a few people in a group have bothered to read material suggested or if participants allow personal problems between members of the group to "charge the atmosphere" and make it uncomfortable. Your teachers will probably be all too aware if this seems to be the case and it may be helpful to ask them to find ways to improve group dynamics.

Managing work-experience

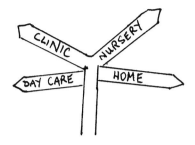

Experience in the workplace is a valuable part of a vocational health and social care course. Some schools and colleges ensure that all students taking the Intermediate GNVQ in Health and Social Care do one or more work placements as part of the course. At the placement, students can develop and practice useful skills, such as **communication** or the **assessment of clients' needs**. Workplace experience can be included in records of achievement and described in job or higher education applications.

Most important of all, the student has the chance to find out at first hand about the career path they are interested in and whether, in the end, it is really what they would like to do.

FINDING A PLACEMENT

It is useful to find out at the beginning of your course, whether your school or college will offer to arrange work-placements for you and whether or not they are a compulsory part of the course. If they are not part of the course you may wish to consider arranging your own relevant work-experience, perhaps on a part-time basis or during holidays. If your college or school arranges the placements, they may still be very happy for you to make suggestions of your own about where you would like to work, especially if you have contacts in that workplace and could set up the placement for yourself.

It is worth bearing in mind that it is often very difficult for teachers and lecturers to find enough suitable placements for their students. Other trainees on professional courses such as social workers, teachers and nurses are often given priority for placements. There are also some workplaces where it would not be safe or advisable to offer experience to younger or less qualified students. Therefore, the more active you are in working with your teachers to find your own placements the more likely it is that you will work somewhere of direct relevance and benefit to you.

Use your local Yellow Pages, library and Citizen's Advice Bureau for names, addresses and telephone numbers of workplaces and organisations within a reasonable travelling distance of where you live. Look for:

- hospitals (think about which **areas** of hospital work would be more likely to offer placements)
- community health clinics
- social services

- Citizen's Advice Bureaux
- public health authorities
- voluntary agencies
- nurseries and play groups
- schools (including special schools, day or residential)
- probation hostels
- day care centres for people with physical or learning disabilities
- residential homes for people with physical or learning disabilities
- day centres for elders
- residential homes for elders
- complementary health practitioners such as osteopaths, chiropractors and homeopaths
- physiotherapists and occupational therapists.

PLANNING THE WORK-PLACEMENT

Length and timing of placement

Your experience of the work–placement will be very different if you, for example, spend four continuous working weeks at the workplace (a block placement) rather than spend a single day a week at the placement throughout the course. The timing of the placement may be out of your control but if you *are* offered a choice it requires careful consideration.

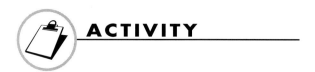

ACTIVITY

1 What do you consider to be the advantages and disadvantages of the two types of work experience arrangements, block and single day each week?
2 On a full time, two year health and social care course, what would you consider to be an adequate length of time to spend in the workplace?

If you are offered more than one work placement it may be helpful to deliberately choose very different sorts of placements so that the greatest range of experience is acquired.

Making practical arrangements

If you can, try to visit the establishment at which you will be working before the official placement begins. Permission to visit may be arranged by your teachers and tutors or you may be expected to arrange this yourself. Permission to visit can be requested by letter or telephone. Be willing to give a concise description of your course, your intended career and what you hope to achieve from the placement.

Confirm in writing when you will make your preliminary visit. Once this is arranged, use this opportunity to meet the staff and to find out:

- How to get there.
- Which key staff you will be working with (try to note down their names)
- The hours you will be working.
- The likely tasks you will be involved in.
- What type of dress will be suitable.
- Practical arrangements, for example, where and for how long you will have lunch.

If you are basing all or part of an assignment on the work-experience placement, take a copy of this and explain the assessment procedure to the person supervising you at the placement. Check with your school or college that the necessary **insurance** has been arranged. This is particularly important if you have set up your own placement.

Making the most of the placement

Many workers in the caring professions are under a great deal of pressure, perhaps because of under staffing, or perhaps because of the nature of the job. It may be an added pressure for them to work with a student. If you observe the following points it will help your working relationship to flourish:

- Find out as much as you can about the placement before you arrive.
- Be punctual.
- Inform your college tutor and your work-experience supervisor of any unavoidable absences but keep these to an absolute minimum.
- Be prepared to work shift–work hours.
- Be co-operative, friendly and helpful. If there does not seem much for you to do, find a moment to ask if you can be given any extra jobs. Use every opportunity to communicate with the patients, clients or service users.
- Treat patients, clients and service users with respect.
- Observe confidentiality
- Show interest by asking questions at convenient times.

Remember! The impression you giver may affect the employer's willingness to offer students placements in the future. It is sometimes the case that, following the placement, students are offered further part-time paid work or even find themselves returning, in the future, for an interview for a full-time post.

Tasks to be carried out prior to placement

To gain the maximum benefit from the work placement it is vital to be well prepared. The following tasks are suggestions to help you with this preparation.

1 Following your preliminary visit, discuss your feelings and reactions with your teachers, tutors and fellow students. The following areas should be covered:
   - Your initial impressions.

- The atmosphere at the placement.
  The patients, clients or service users.
- The staff involved in the care of the patients, clients or service users.
- Issues of confidentiality.
- Your experience of what you can contribute to and will gain from the placement, including how you think the placement could help you acquire the practical and personal skills that you will need in the career you want to follow.

2   It is more than likely, especially if you have already carried out work-experience placements or have other prior or current part of full-time working experience, that you have many positive attributes and skills to offer to the placement. It is important to recognise and be proud of these accomplishments. The ways in which you subsequently develop and add to your "skills profile" at the work-placement can then be noted and will give you valuable information to put into your curriculum vitae or future applications for jobs, training or education.

Use the "Skills Checklist" (Table 10) to carry out a self-appraisal. If there are any areas identified which you feel might cause you some problems at the workplace, make sure that you discuss these with your tutor/teachers so that you can plan strategies for dealing with them before the placement begins.

SKILL	SCORE 1	2	3	4
Ability to respond to instructions.				
Ability to assess when to ask for help.				
Listening skills.				
Ability to take the initiative.				
Ability to work collaboratively.				
Ability to establish relationships.				
Accuracy in practical tasks.				
Good record of punctuality.				
Time management.				
Ability to respond to criticism.				
Ability to present written reports.				
Ability to handle calculations.				
Good attendance record.				
Ability to show enthusiasm and effort.				
Self-confidence.				
Research skills.				

TABLE 10 *Skills checklist for work experience placements.*

The skills checklist can be used for self-appraisal before and after a work experience placement. Score **4** for **very good**, **3** for **good**, **2** for **acceptable** and **1** for **poor** levels of skill.

TASKS TO BE CARRIED OUT IN THE WORKPLACE

Exactly how you use your work-experience will depend partly upon the ways you may be using it to write an assignment, write case-studies or complete a research project. The following written tasks may help you focus on the kinds of information and experience the placement could offer:

1   Keep a diary or log book. In it:
- note activities undertaken each day and the time spent on them.
- record your feelings and reactions to your experiences.

   Describe:
- the **service(s)** provided by your work experience establishment. What service does it offer, and to whom? Is there a hierarchical management or staffing structure in the workplace? Are there different departments? How do the different departments and staff liaise with each other?
- The needs of the **patients, clients** or **service users**.
- the work of the **staff** with whom you come into contact. What are the main qualities/skills they need? What qualifications do they have?

2   If you hope to use the placement to carry out one or more case studies, you should only do this after a preliminary discussion with placement staff as to what aspects of the task are considered to be both permissible and possible. **Confidentiality** and respect for the individual, family or group concerned should be maintained. Once permission for the study has been given you could:
- Use your diary or log book to gather details (such as age, sex, family situation, special interests and abilities, past and current experiences) relevant to the individual(s) or group being studied. Please note that you should never use real names. Use pseudonyms.
- Analyse the role of the institution or service-provider in relation to the individual(s) or group being studied.
- Make notes on the attitudes and feelings that the patients, clients or service users have towards their situation. Reassure the service user that no names will be used in your notes.
- Observe the ways in which staff interact with and influence the patients, clients or service users.
- Examine and record examples of group interactions and dynamics.

3   Investigate and comment on the following aspects of health and safety in your workplace:
- Safety policy and the role and training of first aiders.
- Any actual or potential hazards to staff and patients /clients or service users.
- Any provision of rest or reception areas for patients, clients or service users.

4   Evaluate the role of Information and Communication Technologies in the workplace: how they are used, the tasks they perform and the software employed. Consider tasks being performed (such as filing and report-writing) which could be computerised. Assess the potential and actual value of computers and other communication technologies in the workplace.

5   Keep a note (in your diary or log book) of any issues or questions arising during the work-experience that you would like to discuss with your tutor or other students.

TASKS TO BE CARRIED OUT FOLLOWING THE PLACEMENT

1   Produce an assessment of your own strengths and weaknesses during your placement. Refer back to your skills checklist completed prior to the time spent in the workplace.
- Has your self–appraisal changed?
- Have your career aims changed?
- Have you gained additional skills useful for your intended career? Update your CV and, if possible, plan strategies for overcoming any remaining areas of weakness or "skills gaps".

2   Give an oral presentation of your work experience to other students. This should include:
- Your own role and tasks — what you were required to do.
- The challenges and problems you faced.
- An assessment of what you have learned and what personal development you feel has taken place.

3   Try to ensure that you have a chance to talk informally to your tutor or teachers about the placement. You should also have the chance to receive more formal assessment and "feedback" on your work from your placement supervisor and colleagues and your tutor and teachers. To this end…

4   Write a letter of thanks to the employer(s) concerned and:

5   Prepare a written evaluation of the placement:
- What aspects were most or least satisfactory?
- What changes would you make in the workplace if you could?
- Would you recommend the placement to another student?

The Key Skills Qualification

Each Key Skill is described in a unit that makes it clear what you need to know and be able to to do to meet the standard required. Your school or college should supply you with a copy of the unit descriptions, and will help you to show how you can prove you have achieved the standards required. As a general guideline however, what you **must do** to achieve Level 2 of the Key Skills Qualification is reproduced here.

You must:

Evidence must show you can:

C2.1a

Contribute to a dicussion about a straight forward subject

- make clear and relevant contributions in a way that suite your purpose and situation;
- listen and respond appropriately to what others say; and
- help to move the discussion forward.

C2.1b

Give a short talk about a straightforward subject, using an image.

- speak clearly in a way that suits your subject, purpose and situation;
- keep to the subject and structure your talk to help listeners follow what you are saying; and
- use an image to clearly illustrate you rmain points.

C2.2c

Read and summarise information from **two** extended documents about a straightforward subject. One of the documents should include at lease **one** image.

- select and read relevant material;
- identify accurately the lines of reasoning and main points from text and images; and
- summarise the information to suit your purpose.

C2.3

Write **two** different types of documents about straightforward subjects.

One piece of writing should be an extended document and include at lease **one** image.

- present relevant information in an appropriate form;
- use a structure and style of writing to suit your purpose; and
- ensure text is legible and that spelling, punctuation and grammar are accurate, so your meaning is clear.

FIGURE 14 *Key Skill: Communication What you must do.*

You must:

N2.1

Interpret information from **two** different sources, inclkuding material containing a graph

N2.2

Carry out calculations to do with:
a amounts and sizes;
b scales and proportion;
c handling statistics;
d using formulae

N2.3

Interpret the results of your calculations and present your findings. You must use at least **one** graph, **one** chart and **one** diagram.

Evidence must show you can:

- choose how to obtian the information needed to meet the purpose of your activity;
- obtain the relevant information; and
- select appropriate methods to get the results you need.

- carry our calculations, clearly showing your methods and levels of accuracy; and
- check your methods to identify and correct any errors, and make sure your results make sense.

- select effective ways to present your findings;
- present your findings clearly and describe you rmethods; and
- explain how the results of your calculations meet the purpose of your activity.

FIGURE 15 *Key Skill: Application of number What you must do.*

You must:

IT2.1

Search for and select information for two different purposes.

IT2.2

Explore and develop information, and derive new information, for two different purposes

IT2.3

Present combined information for two different purposes.

Your work must include at least one example of text, one example of images and one example of numbers

Evidence must show you can:

- identify the information you need and suitable sources;
- carry out effective searches; and
- select information that is relevant to your purpose.

- enter and bring together information using formats that help development;
- explore information as needed for your purpose; and
- develop information and derive new information as appropriate.

- select and use appropriate layouts for presenting combined information in a consistent way;
- develop the presentation to suit your purpose and the types of information; and
- ensure your work is accurate; clear and saved appropriately.

FIGURE 16 *Key Skill: Information Technology What you must do.*

Glossary

action plan – a detailed and structured plan for an assignment or piece of work.

analyse – examine in detail: separate into component parts.

assignments – pieces of work set and assessed as part of the requirements of the course.

autonomous learners – students who have become self-reliant.

bibliography – a list of the books referred ton an assignment, essay or other piece.

brain storming – a way of generating ideas before beginning a piece of work.

client – an individual receiving support, treatment or therapy from a health or social care service.

comparison – an analysis of similarities and differences.

conclusion – a summing–up, for example, of ideas, arguments or evidence used in an assignment or essay.

confidentiality – respect for the privacy of any information about a client. It is one of the principles which underpins all health and social care practice.

critical evaluation – where evidence has been used to support judgements or views.

cueing and signal words – words which, in a written or oral presentation, warn of impending and significant changes in the pace, emphasis and order of the content.

curriculum vitae CV – a brief account of one's education and previous occupation often required when applying for a new job.

define – give an exact meaning of a word or concept.

describe – give a written, visual or oral account, as required.

discuss – consider an issue from various points of view.

dyslexia – dyslexia is evident when fluent and accurate word identification (reading) and/or spelling is learnt very incompletely or with great difficulty.

editing – checking a document for errors/making changes or modifications.

evaluation – a retrospective review or reassessment.

feedback – to 'give feedback' has come to mean to make a formal or semiformal response to a piece of work or action.

grading requirements – the criteria which determine the grades awarded for the course.

ICT – Information and Communication Technologies i.e. the use of the Internet or Intra net systems as well as computers, Dictaphones, tape recorders, word processors, hardware and software programs, voice mail, fax, E–mail, CD ROM, telephones, electronic spell checkers etc.

identify – pick out key characteristics or what is most important.

illustrate – give examples to support points made.

Internet – an international computer network linking computers from educational institutions, government agencies, industry and domestic users etc.

interpret – show or make clear the meaning.

introduction – a preliminary section at the beginning of a book or pieced of work.

justify – show good reasons for.

meta cognition – the ability to 'think about thinking'

mind–mapping – a technique used to organise thoughts and ideas in linked key words and pictures. This method can be sued for generating ideas and planning work as well as note–taking and revising.

mnemonic – a device which aids the memory.

motivation – to be stimulated by or interested in something.

multisensory – methods of learning which simultaneously 'tap' more than one sense.

note–taking – a way of summarising points in a text which are relevant to whatever is being studied.

personal organisation — refers to the ways in which an individual plans and manages their daily responsibilities.

portfolio – a collection of the different types of evidence which can show successful completion of the course.

primary sources – information or data gathered at first hand.

prioritising –putting things in order of importance so that the most pressing issues are tackled first.

proof – evidence that something is 'true'

proof–reading – reading through a document for errors.

PQ4R – a reading note–taking method: **P**review, **Q**uestion, **R**ead, **R**eflect, **R**ecite, **R**eview.

reception reading – where reading takes place a steady pace and what is being read is fairly easy to absorb and understand.

records of achievement – a portfolio of educational and personal achievement.

reflective reading – reading which involves thinking about and evaluating what is read.

secondary sources – information or data from the work or research of other people.

service user – an individual using or accessing a social or public service.

skim–reading – the process of running eyes over a text to extract essential or key information.

special assessment concessions – special test arrangements (such as extra time) and/or special consideration (action taken after the examination) in public examinations.

spell–checker – an electronic dictionary.

spider diagrams – a diagrammatic way of representing ideas or information which brings out the main themes and their relationships to each other.

theory – a system of ideas explaining something.

thesaurus – a book that lists words in groups of synonyms (words with similar meanings) and related concepts.

visual thinker – someone who prefers to organise their thoughts in images or patterns.

work experience – time spent in a workplace to gain related experience and knowledge.

Resources
Books

Buzan, T. (1993), *The Mind Map Book*. London: BBC Publications.

Buzan, T. (1995), *Use Your Memory*. London. BBC Books.

Buzan, T. (1996), *Use Your Head*. London. BBC Books.

Cardwell, M (1996), *The Complete A-Z Psychology Handbook*. London Hodder and Stoughton.

Gilroy, D.E. and Miles, T.R. (1996) *Dyslexia at College*. Routledge.

Indge, B. (1997) *The Complete A-Z Biology Handbook*. London, Hodder and Stoughton.

Lawson, T. and Garrod, J. (1996), *The Complete A-Z Sociology Handbook*. London, Hodder and Stoughton.

Mitchell, J.E. (1998), *Student Organiser Pack*, London: Communication and Learning Skills Centre, 131 Homefield Park, Sutton, Surrey, SM1 2DY.

Nortledge, A. (1990), *The Good Study Guide*. Milton Keynes, The Open University.

Richards, J. (1999) *The Complete A-Z Health and Social Care Handbook*. London, Hodder and Stoughton.

SOFTWARE

Type to Learn (Windows, Mac) – teaches students to type while reinforcing spelling, grammar, composition and punctuation skills. Available from Iansyst Tel: 01223 420101

Touch-type, read and spell – specially designed for dyslexic learners by Philip Alexandre Tel: 0181 464 1330.

Touch Type (Windows, Acorn, Mac) see, hear, type from Inclusive Technology Tel: 01457 81970.

Mavis Beacon Teaches Typing – Mindscape. Version 8 English. Available from most high streets stores or Priority House, Charles Av, Maltings Park, Burgess Hill, W. Sussex RH15 9TQ

Wordswork for Windows 3.x/95/98/NT – cost for single person's use £125.00 Distributed by iANSYST Ltd and Brind Arena/Ellen Morgan. Enquiries to sales@dyslexic.com or phone 01223 420101.

Aimed at dyslexic undergraduates, this programme is also useful for students in upper secondary, tertiary and further education and for dyslexic adults wanting to improve their skills before returning to formal study. The programme uses graphics, voice–overs, colour and humour to develop language skills in essay writing, revision, grammar, handwriting, memory, oral presentation, punctuation, reading, spelling, time management and vocabulary building.

textHELP!@Read and Write for Windows 95/98/NT – cost £115 + VAT. Distributed by iANSYST Ltd. FREEphone 08000 1800 45 The White House, 72 Fen Road, Cambridge CB4 1UN Tel 01223 420101 Fax: 01223 42 66 44 sales@dyslexic.com http://www.dyslexic.com

This programme includes an advanced phonetic spell checker, a word prediction facility, homophone support and a log which will record typical spelling errors for future analysis.

Dyslexia and ICT – Building on Success by Sally McKeown (Becta Publications 2000, Becta Bookshop, Milburn Hill Road, Science Park, Coventry CV4 7BR) is a very useful guide to software for dyslexic students.

ORGANISATIONS

British Dyslexia Association
98 London Rd,
Reading RG1 5AU
Helpline 0118 966 8271, Administration 0118 966 2677

The Dyspraxia Foundation,
8, West Alley,
Hitchin, Herts SG5 1EG
Helpline: 01462 454986

Skill (National Bureau for Students with Disabilities)
3rd Floor,
Chapter House,
18–20 Crucifix Lane,
London SE1 3JW
Tel. 0800 3285050

Royal National Institute for the Deaf (RNID)
19–23 Featherstone St.
London EC1Y 8SL
Helpline – voice 0870 6050 123, textphone 0870 6033 007

Royal National Institute for the Blind (RNIB)
224 Great Portland Street
London W1N 6AA
0171 388 1266

Disablement Information and Advice Lines (DIAL UK)
Park Lodge,
St. Catherine's Hospital
Tickhill Road,
Balby, Doncaster
South Yorkshire DN4 8QN
01302 310123

Other

Students with dyslexia, dyspraxia or other disability in full time education may be able to claim a **Disabled Students Allowance**. This is a lump sum with which the student can pay for equipment or services, e.g. to buy a tape recorder and/or photocopying and specialist tuition. For more information about this allowance contact your local Education Authority (if you live in England) and ask for an application form for the allowance. If your school or college has a disability co-ordinator, she or he should also be able to help and advise on how to make a claim.

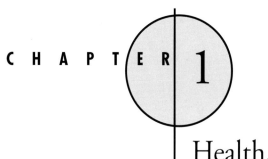

C H A P T E R 1

Health, social care and early years provision

After working through this chapter you should know:

● the main roles of people who work in health and social care and early years – services and the structures within which they function

● the care value base that underpins all health and social care work that is done with clients

● the skills that are needed by people working in the health, social care and early years services

● the basic communication skills that are needed by people working in the health, social care and early years services

In each section, you will find exercises and activities to help you work through the material.

At the end of the chapter, you will find a glossary, references used in the chapter, lists of useful addresses and possible resources you or your teacher could find helpful. Answers to activities, where appropriate, will be found at the end of the Chapter.

Health, social care services and early years services can be divided into four separate divisions (see Figure 1.1).

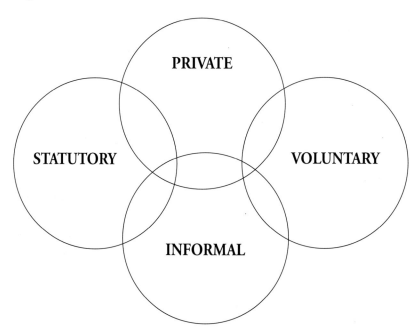

FIGURE 1.1 *The four divisions of health, social care and early years services.*

- Statutory services are funded and provided by central or local agencies. Examples of statutory health services are NHS services including hospitals, school nursing and community nursing. Examples of statutory social care services would be the services provided by the local authority social services department.

- Private services provide a range of services, including private hospitals, private residential homes and private nurseries.

- Voluntary services are provided by voluntary (or non-profit making) organisations that are usually registered as charities and may provide services to particular client groups, e.g. Age Concern provides day centres, Mencap provides a range of services to people with learning difficulties.

- Informal Services are provided outside the other 3 sectors and are usually unpaid. Examples of informal care would be a local church lunch club, a baby sitting group, and relatives caring for older family members.

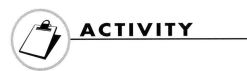

ACTIVITY

Look at the following list and decide which is statutory, voluntary, private or informal.

1 A married daughter looking after her 75 year old mother

2 A GP (general practitioner or family doctor)

3 A Meals on Wheels service

4 A Consultant working in a private hospital
  (see end of Chapter for Answers.)

The National Organisation of the NHS

The White Paper, the *New NHS, Modern Dependable,* was published in 1997 and outlined the plans to modernise the NHS over the next ten years. Many changes have taken place in the organisation of health care, and we will look at some of these in this section.

The Department of Health is the National Government department in charge of the organisation of the Health Service in the UK. With the changes that are taking place in Wales, Scotland and Ireland, these regions will be taking over the control of health in their areas, but the organisation of health is similar in all parts of the UK.

The Secretary of State for Health has overall responsibility for the NHS (See Figure 1.2).

Do you know his/her name?

Figure 1.3 shows how the NHS is divided into regions.

England is divided into 8 regions.

Wales is divided into 4 regions.

Scotland is divided into 15 Health Boards (Figure 1.4).

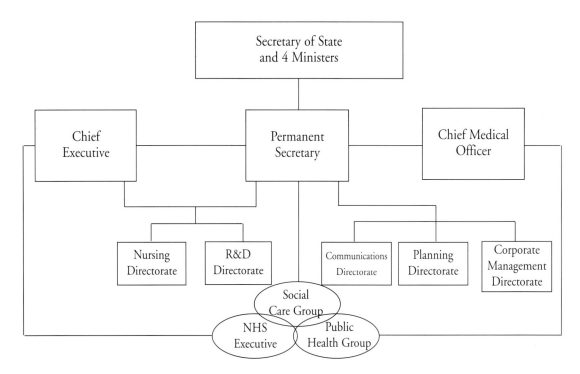

FIGURE 1.2 *Organisation chart of the department of health.*

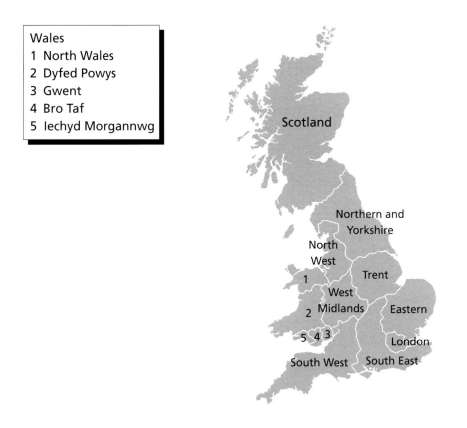

FIGURE 1.3 *Diagram showing regional boundaries for NHS in England and Wales 1999.*

Northern Ireland is divided into 4 Health and Social Care Boards (Figure 1.4).

As you can see the regions are very different. Some areas are highly populated with towns and cities, other regions are in remote rural areas. Each region has a Regional Health Authority that is responsible for the NHS in the Region. Each Region is further divided into District Health Authorities. Figure 1.5 shows the organisation of the NHS at regional level.

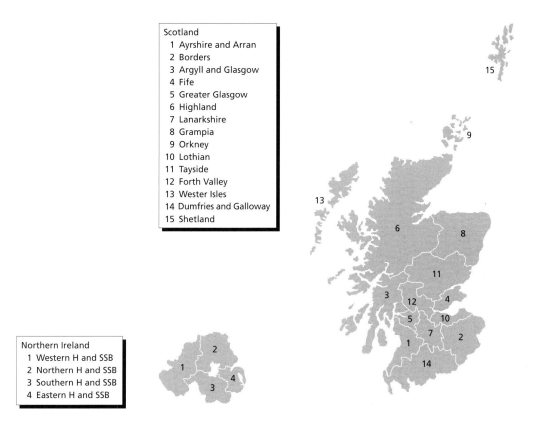

FIGURE 1.4 *Boundaries for Health boards in Scotland and Health & Social Services boards in Northern Ireland (April 1999)*

The full map of regional and health authorities is available on the following web site: www.doh.gov.uk/pub/docs/doh/romap.pdf Using the internet, see if you can identify your region on it.

The Role of the District Health Authority

1   To assess the health needs of the population
2   To draw up a plan to meet those needs (under the New NHS organisation this will be in the form of a Health Improvement programme (or HImP) that is developed in partnership with the Local Authority and the Voluntary Sector)
3   To allocate funding to Primary Care Groups

As you can see from Figure 1.5 DHAs work together with Primary Care Groups, NHS Trusts and Local Authorities. Each DHA covers a population of about 500,000 people.

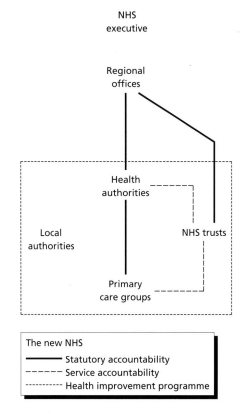

FIGURE 1.5 *The organisation of the NHS at regional level.*

DHAs have to produce an Annual Report. This is a public document that should be available in local libraries but you could phone the DHA and ask for a copy to be sent to you.

The Annual Report gives information about:

● the numbers of GPs in the area

● the numbers of dentists

● the numbers of opticians

● the numbers of community pharmacists

In each year in a typical DHA there are:

● 5 million prescriptions written

● 62,000 NHS eye tests

● 78,000 immunisations and vaccinations

● 102,00 acute hospital admissions

● 9000 babies delivered

(ref: Merton, Sutton and Wandsworth Health Authority Annual Report 1999)

Primary Care Groups

As part of the New NHS, Primary Care Groups (PCGs) were set up in April 1999. There are 481 PCGs, covering populations of 46,000 to 257,000. Groups of practices and GPs are grouped together. Each PCG has a Board which consists of the following members:

- 4 – 7 GPs (depending on the size of the area)
- 1 or 2 community nurses
- 1 Social services representative
- 1 Lay member (a patient who lives in the area)
- 1 Health Authority Non–Executive Director

The Board is led by a Chief Executive. The lay member is on the Board to make sure that the voice of the patients is heard.

FUNCTIONS OF THE PCG

1 To improve the health of the community, making sure that all local people have access to NHS services
2 To develop and improve Primary Care
3 To commission (order and pay for) services that meet the needs of their patients

PCGs operate at 4 levels (figure 1.6).

Level 4	Become trusts. Accountable to the Health Authority but providing care (employing staff) as well as Commissioning Services
Level 3	Become established as free-standing bodies accountable to the Health Authority for commissioning care.
Level 2	Take some responsibility for managing the budget for healthcare, acting as part of the Health Authority.
Level 1	Act in support of the Health Authority in Commissioning Care for it's population, acting in an advisory capacity.

FIGURE 1.6 *The 4 levels of operation of PCGs.*

Over time it is expected that PCGs will become free standing Trusts, which means that they will employ staff (nurses, and other community health workers) as well as commission services.

In this section we have mentioned these terms that we need to clarify:

- **Primary and Secondary care**
- **Primary health care**

This is health care that takes place in the community through the GP, district nurse, practice nurse, Health Visitor, CPN (Community Psychiatric nurse) and other members of the Primary Health Care Team (PHCT). It does not include hospital services.

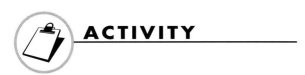

ACTIVITY

Visit your local GP surgery or Health Centre and find out the range of services provided.

Secondary Care

Health care that takes place in hospital. Patients are referred to hospital by their GP except when they refer themselves to Accident and Emergency (A and E) or to the GUM clinic (Genito Urinary Medical clinic for sexually transmitted diseases).

With the development of NHS Direct and NHS Walk In Centres, there may be changes in how referrals are made in the future.

Tertiary Services

Health care that takes place in specialist hospitals, for example cardiac (heart) units, cancer or orthopaedic specialist hospitals.

NHS Trusts

NHS HOSPITAL TRUSTS

Under the 1990 NHS and Community Care Act, hospitals became self governing trusts. This meant they were able to do the following:

- buy, own and sell land and services
- develop their own management systems
- employ their own staff and set out their own terms and conditions of employment (they also used outside companies for cleaning and catering services)
- raise money through developing private patients services, renting out shops in the hospital, car park charges and other ways of raising income

Hospital Trusts have to produce an Annual Report which provides statistics on numbers of patients treated, length of waiting lists, as well as planned developments.

It may be useful if you look at a copy of a hospital trust report. They should be in your local library, or else you can obtain one directly from the hospital.

NHS COMMUNITY TRUSTS

Community Trusts have developed in order to deliver specialist services in the Community. Figure 1.7 shows the services offered by a Community Trust.

South West London Community **NHS**
NHS Trust

Services for Adults
Chiropody, dental services (for people who cannot get treatment within the general dental service) district nursing, HIV/AIDS services, sexual health and family planning, specialist nursing, speech and language therapy, stroke rehabilitation, wheelchair services.

Services for Children and Young People
Child protection, chiropody, continence services, dental services, early years screening, family planning, health visiting, HIV/AIDS services, immunisation and vaccination, liaison work with local authorities, school nursing, special needs services, speech and language therapy, audiology, community paediatric service.

Services for Older People
Continuing and short-term nursing care for clients with assessed high levels of need, respite care, community based health care, hospital home.

Services for People with Learning Disabilities
Residential care, day care, short-term health care, respite care, community services, specialist services (e.g. for clients with challenging behaviour), mental health services.

FIGURE 1.7 *Community Trust Services.*

As you can see the following people are offered services:

- Adults
- Children and Young People
- Older People
- People with Learning Disabilities

MENTAL HEALTH SERVICES

Because of the specialist care needed for people with mental health problems Mental Health Trusts have been developed that link hospital and community care for their patients. CPNs (Community Psychiatric Nurses) are part of the outreach team that develops services such as day centres and drop in centres for patients, as well as providing a 24 hour service in the community.

DAY SURGERY

Because of changes in technology, many hospitals offer day surgery for routine operations such as removal of wisdom teeth, removal of cataracts and other minor operations that require a general anaesthetic. More GPs are offering minor surgery in their practices. This means that the numbers of beds needed in hospital for longer stay patients have gone down.

	1982	1994/95	% CHANGE
No. of beds	143,535	108,000	–39%
No. of inpatient cases	4,412,000	5,662,000	+28%
No. of day cases	684,500	2,433,000	+255%

FIGURE 1.8 *Changes in bed use 1982 – 1994/95.*

Ref. Wellards NHS Handbook 1999/2000

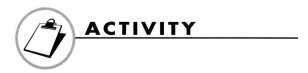 **ACTIVITY**

Look at Figure 1.8.

1   **What is the difference in bed numbers between the years? (See end of Chapter for Answers.)**

2   **How many more inpatients in 1994, compared to 1982?**

3   **What is the difference in day cases between 1994/5 and 1982?**

EMERGENCY SERVICES

NHS hospitals provide emergency services 24 hours a day. On entry to A and E, you will be seen immediately by a triage nurse who will assess your need for treatment.

With the development of NHS Direct it is hoped that the use of A and E for minor problems will be reduced, and that people will either self–care, see their GP or consult a pharmacist.

Recent Developments in the NHS

NHS DIRECT

This is a 24–hour help line staffed by nurses who will give advice on the telephone. NHS Direct has 17 call centres which cover two thirds of the UK. It will cover all of England by the end of the year 2000, and it will also be introduced to Wales and Scotland in the same year.

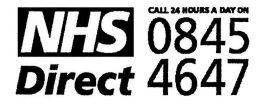

CASE STUDY ● CASE STUDY ● CASE STUDY ● CASE STUDY ● CASE STUDY ● CASE STUDY ●

Ectopic pregnancy

Lisa, a 28 year old mother of three, was suddenly gripped with abdominal pain. She was reluctant to call her GP. Assuming it was a violent stomach upset, she took some pain killers, not even realising she was pregnant. Her partner contacted NHS Direct and the nurse recognised the danger instantly. Within minutes of the call, Lisa was on her way to hospital and undergoing emergency surgery for ectopic pregnancy (the embryo is in the fallopian tube instead of in the womb, and is a serious emergency).

Nurses on NHS Direct can advise callers to self care, see the pharmacist or their GP. They can also advise callers to dial 999 or to attend A and E.

The most common symptoms on which advice is sought are listed in Figure 1.9.

ADULTS	CHILDREN
abdominal pain	fever
fever	vomiting
headache	rash
chest pain	diarrhoea
vomiting	cough
breathing difficulty	cold/flu
back pain	abdominal pain
urinary disorder	headache
sore throat	crying baby
cough	head injury
rash	earache
diarrhoea	chicken pox
cold/flu	poisoning – indigestion
dizziness	upper respiratory infection
finger and toe injuries	eczema
vaginal bleeding	bone injury
skin wound problems	ligament/muscle injury
leg pain	finger and toe injuries
	breathing difficulties
	wounds

FIGURE 1.9 *20 most common symptoms on which advice is sought from NHS Direct.*

Source: data from NHS Direct sites, April 1999

NHS Walk In Centres

These centres are being developed in major towns and cities. They are open from 7 a.m. to 10 p.m. for advice and clinical treatment by nurses and doctors.

NHS Internet Service

The web site, www.NHSDirect.nhs.uk was launched in December 1999. This website gives information about the NHS and how to use it. It also includes pages on diseases and their treatment. It is an interactive website that allows users to describe their symptoms and to self diagnose (which could have problems!) Depending on your answers, the user will be advised to self care, see the GP or pharmacist, or phone NHS Direct or 999.

It is hoped that all the new services will help people decide on the most appropriate type of treatment and take the burden off the A and E departments.

PRIVATE SECONDARY SERVICES

Private hospitals are an alternative to NHS Secondary care. Private hospitals receive most of their income from payments by patients, either directly or else through private health insurance. Some private hospitals offer their own insurance schemes. Private hospitals offer a range of services in addition to out patient, and in–patient surgical and medical care.

Word check:

Medical care – health care using drugs, physiotherapy and non invasive treatment

Surgical care – includes surgical operations

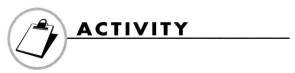 **ACTIVITY**

If you have a private hospital in your area, try to visit it and find out the range of services it offers.

Private Accident and Emergency Care

A private alternative to NHS A and E opened in 1999 (see Figure 1.10). Many people prefer to pay and not have to wait to be seen in an NHS department where the wait can be as long as 3 hours.

Private Primary Care

In some areas there are still private doctors seeing patients. Other private care includes Private Walk In Centres which have developed in airports and railway stations. They offer treatment, advice and travel immunisation.

Welcome to Britain's first private A&E, where six stitches cost £45. So would you pay to jump the queues in casualty?

Imagine it's saturday night and you're in your local casualty – you've hurt your finger, and you are facing a long painful wait surrounded by vomiters, drunks and bleeding children. If you knew you could nip down the road, be whisked through a pleasant (deserted) waiting area, into the arms of a calm, fully-trained doctor or nurse – at a price – would you do it? For most people, the answer to this is yes, depending on the cost. Those made of sterner principles (or with no money) might say "never". But what if it was you four-year-old daughter with the wound.

FIGURE 1.10 *Report on the opening of Britain's first private A and E at Byfleet, Surrey.*

ALTERNATIVE THERAPISTS

These are private services offered in the community. Therapies include:

- Homeopathy
- Osteopathy
- Chiropractic
- Acupuncture

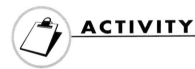 **ACTIVITY**

Use your local phone directory or Yellow Pages, to find the types of alternative therapies that are available in your area.

STATUTORY SOCIAL CARE

The Government finances a range of statutory services, through the local authorities. Money is spent by the local authority on:

- education
- social services

Figure 1.11 shows that most of the money spent by the local authority, is spent on education.

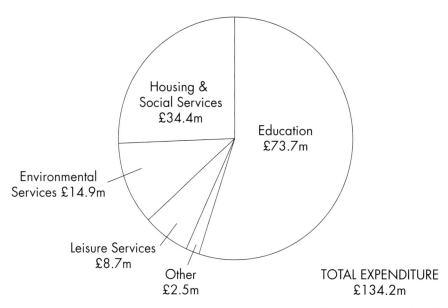

Ref London Borough of Sutton 1998/99 Report

FIGURE 1.11 *Local Authority expenditure.*

The local authority receives money from Central Government, from payment for services and also from the rates that are paid by the local community. Figure 1.12 shows a diagram of a typical Social Services Department.

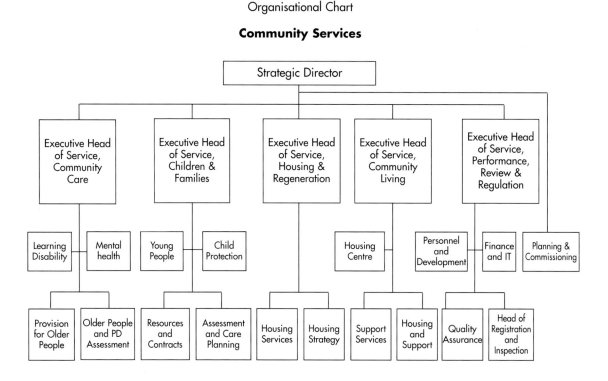

FIGURE 1.12 *Example of a Local Authority Social Services Department.*

There are four main areas of social care provision:

- **Residential care** – care provided in residential homes
- **Domiciliary care** – care provided in the client's own home
- **Day care** – care provided at special centres in the community
- **Field work** – care provided by social workers who care for particular client groups

These client groups are:

- Children and Families
- Older People
- People with Learning Difficulties
- People with Mental Health problems
- People with Drug and Alcohol problems
- People with AIDS and HIV
- Refugees
- Homeless people

Services provided by Social Services include the following:

- assessing needs – providing personal help
- social work
- day care facilities
- residential and respite care facilities
- occupational therapy
- rehabilitation
- supplying specialist equipment
- an emergency service, 24 hours a day, 365 days a year
  Access to social care is through referral and assessment (see diagram 1.1).

MODERNISING SOCIAL SERVICES

This Government Paper was published in 1998. Many people felt that Social Services needed review. There had been scandals involving abuse in residential homes and children's homes, and many people did not receive the help they required when they needed it because of communication difficulties within the organisation, and between the health service and the social services. In addition, the type of social care you received was different in different parts of the country. Local Authorities can decide how much they charge for services and what they should provide.

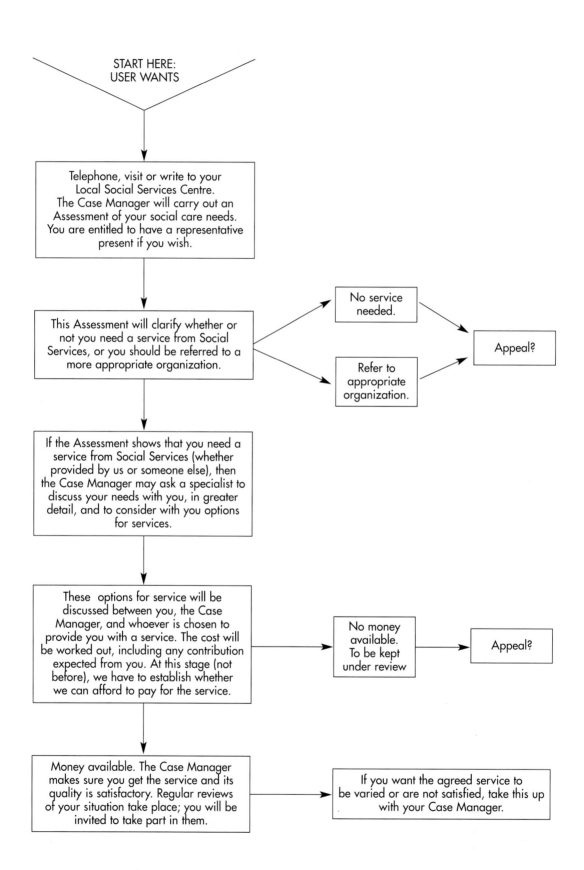

DIAGRAM 1.1 *The assessment procedure carried out by Social Services.*

Word check

- **Duty** – this means that the local authority has to provide the service
- **Power** – means that the local authority can offer this service if it chooses

Examples of services the social services has a duty to provide include:

- an initial assessment of need – this is a free service
- housing for people with mental health problems who have been discharged from hospital

Examples of services the social services may choose to provide include:

- home care facilities

The social services provides some services itself, but nowadays social services buy these services from private or voluntary organisations.

PRIVATE SERVICES

Residential homes

Few residential homes are now owned and run by social services. Most residential homes are private establishments and the local council has a contract with the home to pay for the care of residents. The council will not pay for very expensive homes.

Home care

Many private agencies offer to do shopping and cleaning for clients. The client can either arrange for the service, directly with the agency, or the local council will have a contract with the agency and charge the client for the service.

Voluntary Services

Many voluntary organisations offer a range of services. As the role of the local council has changed from providing services to buying in services, the council may buy its services from a range of organisations.

Since the 1990 NHS and Community Care Act, Voluntary organisations have become providers of a great deal of care.

Diagram 1.2 shows some of the range of services that are provided by voluntary organisations in a London Borough.

● **CASE STUDY** ● **CASE STUDY** ● **CASE STUDY** ● **CASE STUDY** ● **CASE STUDY** ● **CASE STUDY** ●

As part of the preparation for your project we will now look at an example of a Voluntary organisation, from the historical and national perspective and then at a local group.

EXAMPLES OF VOLUNTARY SERVICES FOR DIFFERENT CLIENT GROUPS

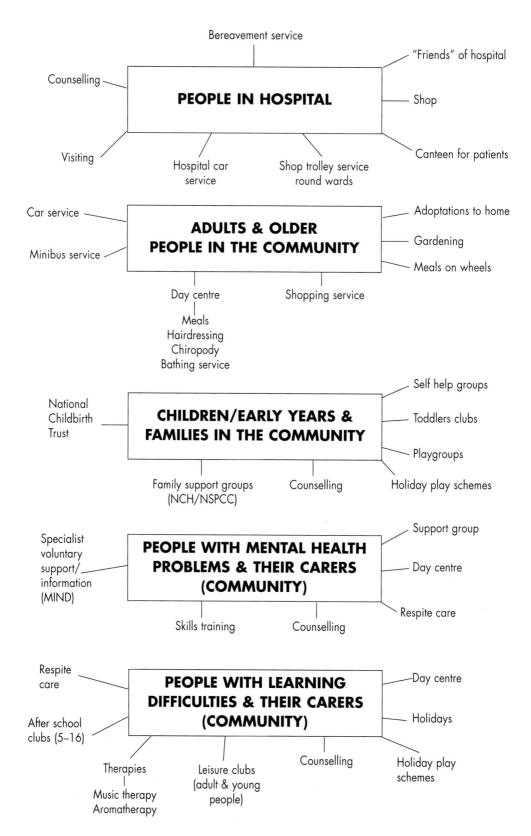

DIAGRAM 1.2 *Examples of voluntary services for different client groups.*

Case Study of a National Voluntary Organisation

Mencap

In November 1946, a young mother with a mentally handicapped child wrote to the "Nursery World" about her problems. Another young mother, Judy Fryd, responded through the column of the magazine and as a result many mothers contacted the magazine and the Association of Backward Children was founded. Members of the group received newsletters and advice, and regional groups were set up throughout the UK. By 1955 there were 167 local groups and the name of the organisation was changed to the National Society for Mentally Handicapped Children. In 1960, World Mental Health Year was celebrated and the Mental Health Act of 1960 abolished the terms mental defective, idiots, imbeciles and feeble–minded. In the 1970s many of the large institutions for people with a mental handicap were closed and the patients were discharged into the community. In 1980 the Society changed its name again to The National Society for Mentally Handicapped Children and Adults (or Mencap).

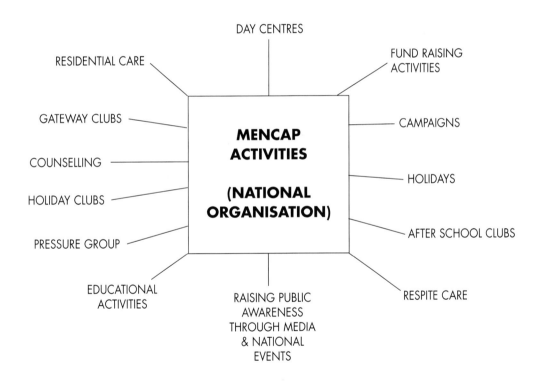

FIGURE 1.13 *Services provided by Mencap.*

With more people of all ages with mental handicap coming into the community, Mencap developed a range of services. (See Figure 1.13) As well as providing services for people with mental handicap (or learning difficulties as it is now called)Mencap is an Action group, trying to influence government policy and also to give information to the general public so that prejudice against people with learning difficulties is reduced. Mencap manages more than 600 homes where adults can live with support. It also provides flats and other accommodation with 24 hour support for the residents.

It has a National College which provides training in life, social and practical skills for people aged 16–25, and other educational projects. It provides an employment service supporting people as they go into work. It has set up a national system of Gateway clubs that provide leisure activities. It offers respite care, counselling, advice and information for families.

(ref: Our Concern the Story of the National Society for Mentally Handicapped Children and Adults. 1946 – 1980.)

Word Check

Learning disability can be defined as a life long condition which results from damage to the brain, before, during or after birth or from genetic or chromosome factors (e.g. Down's syndrome).

● CASE STUDY ● CASE STUDY ● CASE STUDY ● CASE STUDY ● CASE STUDY ● CASE STUDY ●

Local Mencap group

Sutton Mencap was set up to promote the wellbeing of people with a learning disability, their families and carers. The group has recently moved into a refurbished centre near to the shopping centre which is used for a range of services.

Each week, Sutton Mencap has a range of activities. These include:

Saturday play care – *a club that runs during term time offering stimulating play for children and young people aged 5 – 19, and giving families a break 68 people use this service*

After school clubs – *offers play and tea for children aged 5 to 16*

Holiday Play scheme – *offers Activities and outings for 5 to 19 year olds*

Integrated Play Scheme – *during term time, offers 5 to 14 year olds the chance to mix with mainstream children from local schools at the centre*

Stars Unlimited – *a dance and music group for young adults*

Young Adult group – *organises leisure activities*

Carers group

Mencap is represented on a range of local committees. Like the National organisation it is both a campaign group and a support group. It has a local newsletter, organises a range of fund raising activities. At the moment it has 30 volunteers who help in a variety of ways.

● CASE STUDY ● CASE STUDY ● CASE STUDY ● CASE STUDY ● CASE STUDY ● CASE STUDY ●

Local Mencap group (continued)

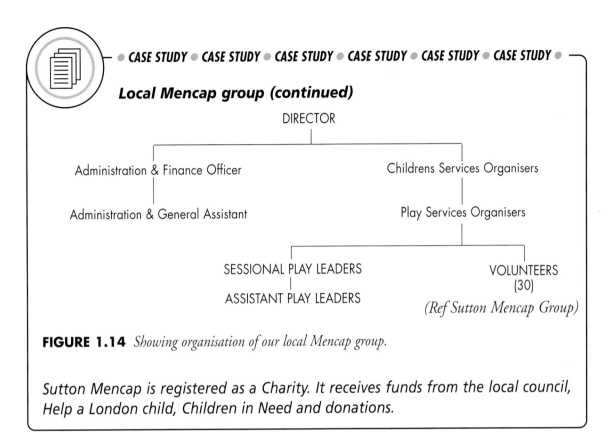

FIGURE 1.14 *Showing organisation of our local Mencap group.*

Sutton Mencap is registered as a Charity. It receives funds from the local council, Help a London child, Children in Need and donations.

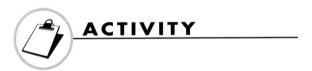

ACTIVITY

A useful book called The Charities Digest (published by Waterlow) gives details of national and local charities in the U. K. It is available in most libraries. Try to obtain a copy and look at the range of charities in health and social care that are listed. Using your local library find out what local groups you have in your area, what groups of people they help, and how they are organised. Perhaps you might arrange to do some voluntary work as part of your work experience.

Many voluntary organisations started off as small local groups and then became national organisations. Volunteers are essential if local groups are going to be able to succeed.

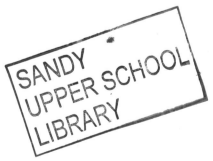

● *CASE STUDY* ● *CASE STUDY* ● *CASE STUDY* ● *CASE STUDY* ● *CASE STUDY* ● *CASE STUDY* ●

The Weekend Break Project is a local voluntary group that was set up to give the carers of people with Alzheimers Disease or dementia a break on Saturdays and Sundays, and also to provide an enjoyable experience for the clients. As the manager of the group said "Having Alzheimers doesn't mean you can't enjoy yourself !"

It was started in 1991 when the Editor of a local paper had a friend who was diagnosed as having Alzheimers Disease, and he saw the effect the disease had on all the family. Through the paper he launched an appeal that raised £30,000 to open Day Care provision at a local hospital unit. The project was supported by the local centre for Voluntary service and the local authority, and 2 centres are now involved in the project on Saturdays and Sundays. The centres are managed by qualified staff, supported by co-ordinators and volunteers. Volunteers act as drivers, escorts and general helpers.

Funding is provided by the local council, from donations and from fund raising events.

The ages of volunteers range from16 to 75, and they are given basic training when they start. Activities include local outings, as well as parties and entertainment. The centres are open from 9.a.m. to 4 p.m. and meals are provided. Clients are referred to the project through the CPN, the Care manager or the Consultant Psychiatrist. Most of the clients live in their own homes or with a carer. They really enjoy their time at the Centre. None of this work would be possible without the volunteers.

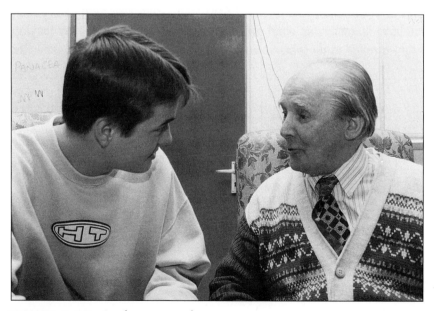

FIGURE 1.15 *A volunteer at a day centre.*

● CASE STUDY ● CASE STUDY ● CASE STUDY ● CASE STUDY ● CASE STUDY ● CASE STUDY ●

Philip is a volunteer with the Project group. He is 17 and studying for his A levels. He wants to be a doctor and he has applied to medical school. He comes every Saturday. He helps with meal times, and plays games with the clients. He goes on outings with the group to help out. He joined the group because he wanted to find out more about Alzheimers. In figure 1.15 Philip is talking to one of the clients.

Stimulation of the person with Alzheimers is very important, and this is done through conversation, games, art work, and reminiscence therapy.

Ashna (18) is another volunteer. She is also hoping to be a doctor. She comes each week, and her main interest is in art and craft work that she does with the group. Because the clients need careful supervision, there is one helper for every four or five people.

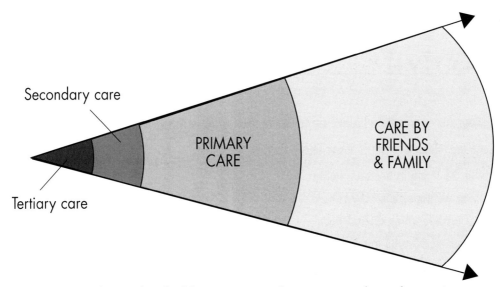

DIAGRAM 1.3 *Showing how health care is moving from tertiary and secondary services to informal care by friends and family.*

INFORMAL CARE

Diagram 1.3 shows how the focus for care has moved away from long stay hospitals into the community. Although the Primary Health Care Team offers health care in the community, family, friends and neighbours offer more and more informal care. Under the 1990 NHS Community Care Act, long stay hospitals were closed and patients moved into the community. People with learning difficulties, physical disability and mental heath problems are now cared for in the community, and in practice this means by the family.

Carers

There are six million carers in the UK, but who are they?

A carer is anyone who is helping to look after a partner, friend or relative who, because of illness, old age or disability may not be able to manage at home without help.

Carers save the Government an estimated £34 billion every year by caring for people at home. Without this informal care, many people would have to live in residential care. It has been estimated that there are 900,000 people who care for someone for more than 50 hours each week.

We will now look at some research carried out by the Princess Royal Trust in a report called *"8 Hours a Day and Taken for Granted"* published in 1998. This report summarises the findings of 7000 questionnaires that were sent to carers centres in the UK, and focuses on the responses of 1,346 carers who care for 8 hours or more each day.

- 63% of these had been caring for more than 5 years
- 94 % are providing medical care but only 33% of these had received any training or guidance of any kind

What is a typical carer?

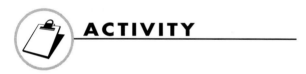

ACTIVITY

These are examples of people who are cared for in their own homes.

For each example, think of who is most likely to care for them.

1 a widow of 88 living in her own home

2 a young man with multiple sclerosis

3 a child of 5 with learning difficulties

4 a married man of 30 who has had a car accident

5 a single woman of 30 recovering from a serious operation

6 a man of 75 living with his wife

These examples show some of the different people that carers look after. Your answers may reflect your views of the role and responsibilities of families, neighbours and friends.

In the following activities you will be able to demonstrate that you can read and understand Charts and Diagrams (Key Skill: Application of Number).

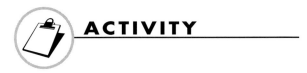

ACTIVITY

If we look at figure 1.16 (showing the relationship to the cared for) we can see that family relationships are important when caring for people:

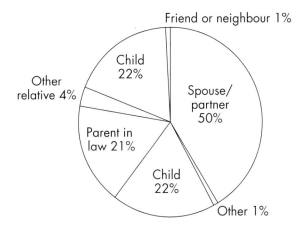

FIGURE 1.16 *Relationship to cared for.*

Look at figure 16 again and answer these questions. (See end of Chapter for Answers.)

1   Which group is most likely to care for someone?
2   Which group is least likely to care for someone?

Many people think that it is mainly older people that are cared for in the community but research shows that there is a wide range of age groups receiving informal care.

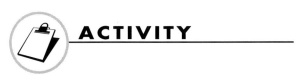

ACTIVITY

Look at Figure 1.17 "Age of Cared for" and answer the following questions (See end of Chapter for Answers.):

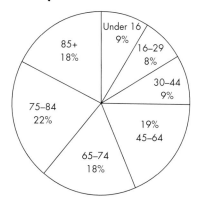

8 hours a day and taken for granted (1998)

FIGURE 1.17 *Age of cared for.*

1   What % of people under 16 are cared for in the home?

2   If you add the % of all age groups under 65 what is the total % cared for at home?

3   How does this compare with the total % over 65 that are cared for at home?

We can see that the % of people over 65 cared for at home is greater than the group under 65, but the difference is not as great as you may have thought.

....

In the last 40 years certain changes have taken place.

These include:

➡   increased life expectancy

➡   an increase in the population that are aged over 75

➡   changes in the treatment of disease and disability which allow people to live longer

➡   shorter stays in hospital for surgery

➡   closure of long stay institutions

What effects do you think these changes will have on carers in the future?

In the past, women did most of the caring in the home for sick and disabled members of the family.

Look at figure 1.18. Is this still the case?

PERCENTAGE OF ADULTS WHO WERE CARERS: BY AGE AND GENDER, 1995–6

Great Britain	Percentages		
	Males	Females	All
16–29	5	6	6
30–44	8	13	10
45–64	17	22	20
65 and over	14	11	13
All aged 16 and over	11	14	13

Source: General Household Survey, Office for National Statistics   *Social trends 1999*

FIGURE 1.18 *Percentage of adults who were carers: by age and gender, 1995–96.*

Why do you think more men are becoming carers now?

Factors that could have brought about change include:

➡   families may not live near each other so that husband and wife support each other more

➡   ideas have changed about what is womens' work and what is mens' work

➡   increased numbers of young carers, including boys under 16

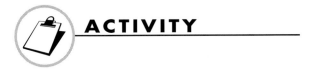

ACTIVITY

What is the age of a typical carer?

Is it?

over 65?

over 40?

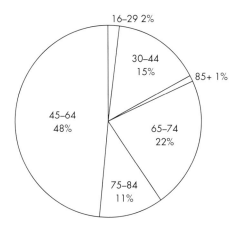

16–29 2%

30–44 15%

85+ 1%

45–64 48%

65–74 22%

75–84 11%

8 hours a day and taken for granted (1998)

FIGURE 1.19 *Age of carer.*

If you look at Figure 1.19 you can see that many carers are under 65.

1 What % are 16 – 45?

2 What % are 16 – 64?

3 How does this compare with the % over 65?
   (See end of Chapter for Answers.)

As we can see a large % of carers are 16 – 64. This means that the caring they do could affect the amount of time they have to spend on education and work. If you are caring for someone at home, how might this affect your work? If you are unable to work because of your caring role, what effects may this have? Many people who are carers find it very tiring, and this affects the work they do. They become stressed and may have to move from full time work to part time work, or give up work altogether. What extra strain could this put on the carer?

➡ low income

➡ no leisure time

➡ no break from caring

Caring can be very time consuming.

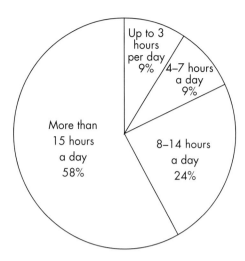

FIGURE 1.20 *Hours caring each day.*

If we look at Figure 1.20 "Hours Caring Each Day", we can see that 58% of carers aged 16+ spend more than 15 hours caring. If there are only 24 hours in a day, this doesn't leave much time for doing other things.

What does caring involve?
Caring could be:

➡ helping someone get up in the morning and to bed at night

➡ cooking a meal and helping them eat it

➡ helping someone have a bath and use the toilet

	NEVER	**OCCASIONALLY**	**REGULARLY**
1 Providing help with dressing	4%	21%	75%
2 Providing help with washing and bathing	5%	18%	75%
3 Providing help with shaving and/or cutting nails	10%	15%	75%
4 providing help with using the toilet	16%	26%	59%
5 Providing help with food and drink	8%	14%	78%
6 Providing help with walking	10%	19%	71%
7 Providing help with moving around the house	12%	26%	62%

TABLE 1.1 *What do carers do?*

Look at Table 1.1

You can see that seven areas of care are identified here. If you look at the 'regularly provided' column, you can see that carers do a great deal of personal care, such as washing, dressing and giving help with meals. Why do you think the categories 4 and 7 are lower than the others? Possibly this could be if a person needs help with mobility and toileting; it may be that they have a high level of need and that residential care is more appropriate for them.

In this section we have looked at carers over 16, but recent research shows that there may be many young carers under 16.

What is the age of the youngest carer?

➡ 14, 12, 10, 8, 6?

The youngest carer known to a carers centre was 6.

In a recent study "Too much to take on" (1999) 20 young carers groups were questioned about caring and bullying. 240 questionnaires were completed. If you look at Table 1.2 you can see the age range of young carers.

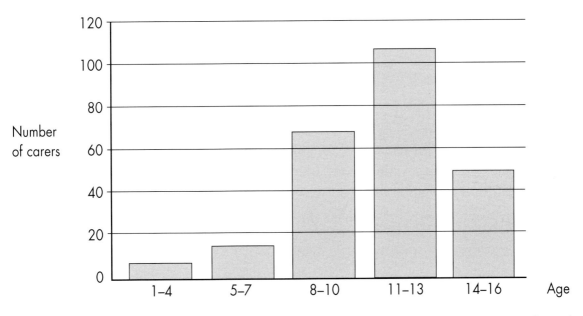

(from "Too Much to Take On" (1999) Princess Royal Trust)

TABLE 1.2 *Age of young carers.*

44% of young carers are aged 11 – 13. This can be a difficult time for young carers as they are changing schools and making new friends. 35% of young carers are 10 or under and this means they are taking on a lot of responsibility at a very young age.

GENDER

More young carers are female. This reflects the older male/female carer split. Table 1.3 shows the relationship of the young carer to the person they are looking after. Describe the main patterns of the Table.

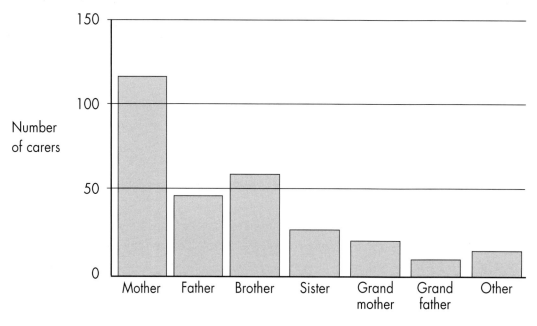

Too Much to Take On" 1999 Princess Royal Trust

TABLE 1.3 *Relationship of the young carer to the person looked after.*

Primary carer

This is the only person providing care, and puts a great deal of pressure on a young person. 16% of young carers in the survey were the primary carer, of the 16 %, 28% were 10 years old or less. Young carers who are primary carers are more likely to care for someone with a physical disability (32%) or a mental health problem (21 %).

Support for young carers

33% of the young carers' teachers did not know they were looking after someone. Many young carers did not tell their friends that they are carers as they felt they would be laughed at and no–one would want to be friends with them. They tried to keep their caring role a secret.

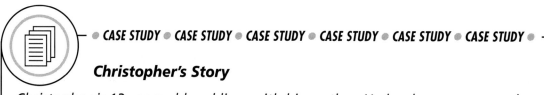

● CASE STUDY ● CASE STUDY ● CASE STUDY ● CASE STUDY ● CASE STUDY ● CASE STUDY ●

Christopher's Story

Christopher is 13 years old and lives with his mother. He has been a carer as long as he can remember. He looks after his mother who needs continuous care, as she has multiple health problems, including epilepsy. Although home carers visit to help with his mother's personal care, they are not there all the time. Paul helps with the household chores and cooking.

● CASE STUDY ● CASE STUDY ● CASE STUDY ● CASE STUDY ● CASE STUDY ● CASE STUDY ●

Christopher's Story (continued)

His mother gets lonely during the day, so he does not like to leave her alone after school and at weekends he helps her with personal care and toileting, although he still feels awkward doing these tasks. His mother has regular epileptic fits which can be quite frightening. Christopher often has to dial 999 and get an ambulance to take his mother to A and E. Each time they had to wait several hours.

Christopher finds he is getting behind with school work. He is always tired because of his caring role and he is always "on call" so it is difficult to relax, look at TV or read a book. He feels the odd one out at school. He has few friends as he finds it difficult to bring them home. He feels embarrassed when school friends see him pushing his mother in a wheel chair. He cannot stay behind at school to play football, because he worries about his mother. He has been bullied verbally by boys calling him names. Sometimes he feels very depressed and frustrated.

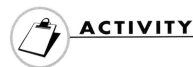

ACTIVITY

Read Christopher's Story.

● **What needs does he have and how could these be met?**

Here is a list of Christopher's problems:

● **Bullying at school**
● **Falling behind with school work**
● **Feeling tired all the time**
● **Coping with the idea his mother is going to die**
● **No time for hobbies and leisure activities**
● **Dealing with epileptic fits**
● **Lack of friends and support**
● **Bullying**

Can you think of possible solutions?

Research shows that 79% of young female carers have been bullied at school, and that 60% of young male carers have experienced bullying. These young people suffered verbal, physical and emotional abuse, and many truanted from school as a result.

Many schools have an Anti Bullying Policy.

What else could be done to help people like Christopher?

Support for Young Carers

Young carers should be identified and assessed for their needs. Only 11% of young carers have been assessed. Teachers should be aware of children who are carers and provide additional support. Young Carers projects are run at Carers Centres and provide activities including painting and outings, as well as counselling, support and advice.

The main jobs in Health and Social Care and Early Years Services

STAFF GROUP	ENGLAND	SCOTLAND	WALES	N. IRELAND	UNITED KINGDOM
Hospital medical staff	52,650	7,080	3,170	2,790	65,6920
Nursing & midwifery staff (inc. students)	332,870	51,470	23,420	18,150	425,910
Other clinical staff	249,710	33,890	18,360	20,070	322,030
All staff	753,610	105,730	52,980	46,046	958,380

FIGURE 1.21 *NHS staff numbers 1999.*

Source: Wellards NHS Handbook 1999/2000

The NHS is one of the largest employers. Figure 1.21 shows the numbers of people employed in the health service. Within the statutory Health and Social Care services in the UK, it is estimated that more than 1 million people are in paid employment.

Within the health and social care sectors, there are those staff who deliver care directly and those whose work is more indirectly involved with care.

Examples of direct care include:
nurse, doctor, social worker, care assistant, nursery nurse

Examples of indirect care include:
clinic clerk, receptionist, cleaner

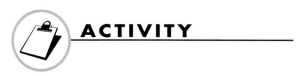 **ACTIVITY**

Look at the following examples of jobs and decide whether they are direct care or indirect care:

- **hospital porter**
- **health visitor**
- **practice manager**
- **practice nurse**
- **chiropodist**

THE DIFFERENCE BETWEEN HEALTH CARE AND SOCIAL CARE

People who work as health workers usually look after patients who have health related problems or conditions. People who work in social care are usually dealing with clients who have a range of personal and social needs. Remember Figure 1.7 which showed the range of services offered by social Services.

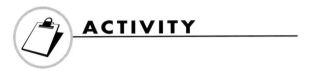 **ACTIVITY**

Look at the following list of jobs and decide which is a health care job, and which is a social care job:

- **Health Visitor**
- **District nurse**
- **Dentist**
- **Pharmacist**
- **Social Worker**
- **Care assistant**
- **Occupational therapist**
- **Community Psychiatric Nurse**
- **Housing officer**

Most of these jobs fit easily into either health care or social care. Two are problematic:

Occupational therapists are employed by social services to assess the needs of people in their homes and the physical support they may need (bath rails, commodes, walking aids) However they can also be employed in hospitals to encourage people to do practical skills and as part of therapeutic treatment in the case of people with mental health problems. The Community Psychiatric Nurse is another example of a job that does not fit easily into either health or social care as although the CPN has a nursing qualification, he or she also provides emotional support.

OCCUPATIONAL AREAS IN HEALTH AND SOCIAL CARE

Before we start to look at the main jobs in health and social care, we need to be aware of the different sectors of employment.

The main categories are divided up as follows:

1　Medicine
2　Nursing
3　Community Services
4　Social Work
5　Child care

6   Professions allied to Medicine (PAMS)

7   Administration and support work

Within each of these groups, there tends to be a common core of training followed by specialist training. For example, all doctors follow a standard medical training and those who choose to specialise in general practice complete additional training. Hospital Play specialists have usually completed their Diploma in Nursery Nursing before they complete the hospital play specialist course.

Main jobs in Health
MEDICINE

Entry into medical school training is very competitive and applicants must have good grades at A level. The training lasts for 5 years. After training the doctor spends at least a year as a junior hospital doctor. After this period doctors take additional training in order to become a specialist in their chosen area of practice.

● **CASE STUDY** ● **CASE STUDY** ● **CASE STUDY** ● **CASE STUDY** ● **CASE STUDY** ● **CASE STUDY** ●

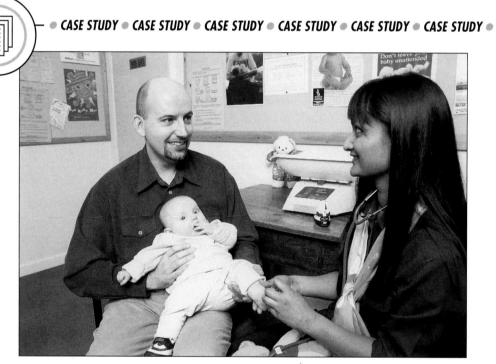

FIGURE 1.22 *A GP consultation.*

Salma is a GP in a busy South London practice. She is married with a young child. Salma took a specialist GP training course after her initial time as a junior doctor. She has a particular interest in paediatrics (children's medicine) and she attends the local children's hospital training sessions. She is also interested in recent developments in drugs and she is on the prescribing sub-committee of her local PCG Board. Salma has three partners at her practice, and she and her colleagues take it in turns to work on Saturdays.

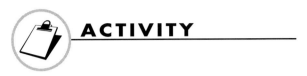

ACTIVITY

Being a GP can be very demanding. Although many of the patients you see can have routine problems that are relatively easy to treat, you can also be faced with emergency situations that need instant decisions. You can also see patients who are extremely anxious, patients who are dying. It has been estimated that GPs can write up to 300 prescriptions a week and they can also see up to 20 people in one session at the surgery.

Diagram 1.4 shows a list of qualities that have been identified as necessary for people working in health and social care. Which 10 qualities would be most important in the role of the GP?

1 Tact	**18** Reliable
2 Sympathy	**19** Trustworthy
3 Firmness	**20** Punctual
4 Kindness	**21** Neat writing
5 Able to work as part of a team	**22** I.T. skills
6 Able to work independently	**23** Maths skills
7 Smart appearance	**24** Get in with all ages
8 Likes children	**25** Willing to work shifts
9 Physical strength	**26** Willing to work long hours
10 Strong hands	**27** Care about cleanliness
11 Good health	**28** Patient
12 Well spoken	**29** Prepared for a long period of
13 Tall	training
14 Confident	**30** Respects others
15 Sense of humour	**31** A good listener
16 Friendly	**32** Telephone skills
17 Efficient	

DIAGRAM 1.4 *The importance of personality skills and health related to jobs in health and social care.*

NURSING AS A CAREER

At the moment entry into the Diploma of Nursing requires applicants to have 5 GCSEs or the Advanced GNVQ in Health and Social Care. Once students are accepted onto the Diploma, they follow a Common Foundation programme for 18 months and then they specialise into one of the following Branches:

- Adult Nursing
- Mental Health
- Learning Difficulties
- Child Health

In September 2000, some colleges will be developing a Diploma with a 1 year Foundation programme. Some students may decide they want to do the degree in nursing. Many nurses who are working in the hospital or community at the moment have completed additional training courses. In this section we will look at some of the jobs in community nursing.

● *CASE STUDY* ● *CASE STUDY* ● *CASE STUDY* ● *CASE STUDY* ● *CASE STUDY* ● *CASE STUDY* ●

The health visitor

Joyce is a health visitor attached to a busy health centre in South London. This is a day in her working week.

9.00 a.m. *arrive at the health centre. Check the post and also messages that have been left during the night. Phone and arrange visits to mothers of babies who have been discharged from the care of the midwife and are now Joyce's responsibility.*

10.00 – 12.00 *Child development clinic, advising mothers on diet and nutrition, sleeping problems. The details of all babies seen are logged onto the computer.*

12.00 *visit to local mother and baby hostel to advise mothers on baby care. This hostel is run by a local church for single unsupported girls. The girls go into the hostel when they are pregnant, and stay until the baby is 6 months old. During the visit Joyce advises on home safety, and weighs the babies on portable scales. The lunch hour is spent dealing with phone calls, writing up reports, including referral to specialist. Although more work is done nowadays on computer, written records are still used.*

2.00 p.m. *Joyce visits a woman of 75 who has urinary incontinence. During her visit Joyce takes the patients family history, numbers of pregnancies, and tests her urine. Joyce advises her how to avoid infections by drinking a lot of water, and she orders incontinence pads.*

3 p.m. *Joyce calls in on a new mother who has been discharged from the midwife. The health visitor takes over from the midwife at the tenth day.*

3.30 p.m. *Joyce visits a family whose three year old daughter attended A and E with a suspected non-accidental injury. Joyce is the named Health Visitor at the Health Centre for these injuries, and she was contacted by the HV based at the hospital.*

7.30 – 9 p.m. *Joyce runs the parentcraft class for women who are near the end of their pregnancy. Husbands or partners are encouraged to be present.*

During the evening she shows a video showing the birth of a baby, and demonstrates the development of the foetus and the delivery using anatomical models, and visual aids. The class is very lively, with people asking questions.

In this part of the evening she organises the parents into groups and asks them to make a list of their worries about pregnancy and childbirth.

Do you think that Joyce needs different skills from the doctor? Look at the list again in Diagram 1.4 and decide which skills are important.

DISTRICT NURSES

District nurses are trained nurses involved with a wide range of patients. They visit people in their own homes, to give clinical care and to advise on nursing aids and equipment. They will change dressings, give injections and administer other treatment. District nurses provide leadership and support to the nursing team, which may include working with health care assistants, studying for their NVQ (National Vocational Qualification) and liaising with social services. Recent changes mean that District Nurses are now able to prescribe drugs on a limited list once they have completed training.

COMMUNITY PSYCHIATRIC NURSES

CPNs are employed by the Community Mental Health Trust and are concerned with supporting people with mental health problems in the community. However they often work closely with their colleagues in hospital.

> ● *CASE STUDY* ● *CASE STUDY* ● *CASE STUDY* ● *CASE STUDY* ● *CASE STUDY* ● *CASE STUDY* ●
>
> *Pam is a CPN in a busy suburban area. She belongs to a team of 7 CPNs who are specialists in the care of patients with dementia. Although most of her patients are over 65, she also has younger patients who have been diagnosed as having dementia at a younger age. Patients are referred to the Consultant Psychiatrist by their GPs. The Psychiatrist sees them within a short time and then refers them to Pam and her team. Each CPN has a caseload of between 35 and 40 patients. Pam sees her patients in their own home, and there are weekly team meetings to discuss the progress of patients and any problems.*
>
> *Pam likes working in the community. She can work on her own initiative. She enjoys building up a relationship with the families she visits and seeing progress of some of patients. The challenges of the job include the stress caused by staff shortages, (which can increase the work load); making difficult decisions. There is a lot of paperwork. It is hard to say goodbye to patients when they have to go into residential care.*

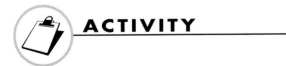

ACTIVITY

We have now looked at several examples of jobs in the community. Are the qualities required for each job the same, or are they different?

Look again at diagram 1.4 and think what qualities are needed for each of the jobs we have discussed in this section.

Community Pharmacist

Another important member of the Community team is the Community pharmacist. For simple complaints, such as coughs and colds, the pharmacist can offer advice. With the development of NHS Direct, more people are being encouraged to talk to their pharmacist to discuss possible treatment. The pharmacist has a wide knowledge of drugs and can advise patients on the side effects they may experience when taking prescribed drugs. Some pharmacists keep records of patient's prescriptions on computer so that they can refer to them. Apart from giving advice and preparing prescriptions, the pharmacist may offer the following services:

➡ Home delivery of drugs to housebound patients

➡ Delivery of oxygen cylinders

➡ Pregnancy testing

➡ Some specialist blood testing for allergies through a private lab

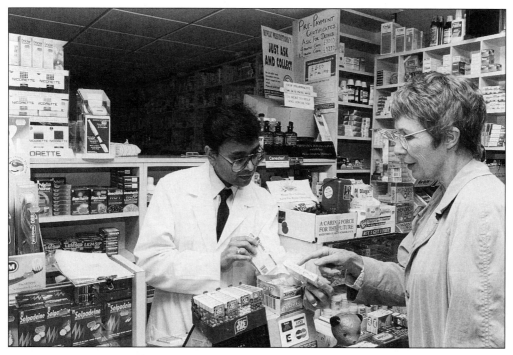

FIGURE 1.23 *Pharmacist at work.*

Dentist

Dentists have a long period of training before they are qualified. Like doctors the training takes 5 years and dentists continue to have regular training once they are in practice, as many of the procedures change and they need to keep up to date. Some dentists have their own private practices but most dentists have a mixture of NHS and private patients. If you have a problem finding an NHS dentist, the District Health Authority will find a dentist for you.

Apart from fillings, replacing broken and damaged teeth and cosmetic dentistry, some dentist specialise in orthodontics, when they treat crooked teeth with appliances that can be fixed or removable. Dentists advise patients about hygiene and dental care.

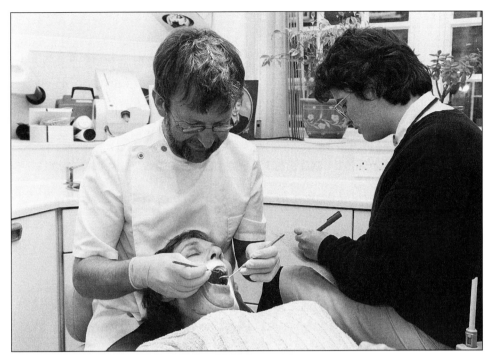

FIGURE 1.24 *Dentist at work.*

Dental nurse

A dental nurse has to have at least 5 GCSEs to be accepted for training. Once qualified, the dental nurse continues to attend training sessions to adapt his/her knowledge.

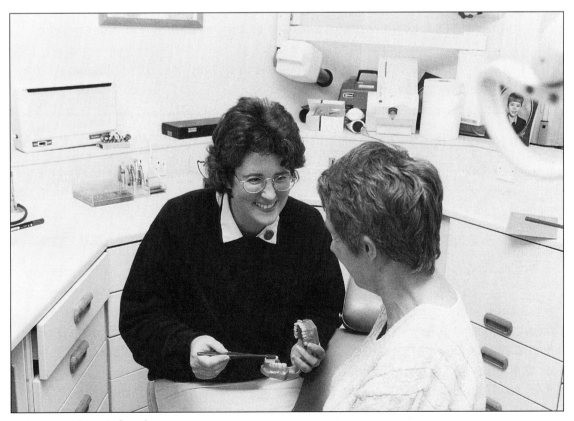

FIGURE 1.25 *A dental nurse.*

Chiropodist

This is another member of the community team. Chiropodists are concerned with maintaining healthy feet. Although many chiropodists are private self–employed practitioners, NHS chiropodists are attached to health centres and can be accessed by referral from a GP or nurse, or by self–referral. Certain groups of people are especially prone to foot problems, older people or people with diabetes. The chiropodist can treat infections of the nails and feet, and advises on foot care.

● CASE STUDY ● CASE STUDY ● CASE STUDY ● CASE STUDY ● CASE STUDY ● CASE STUDY ●

Siobhan is a dental nurse in a busy practice in the South of England.

Her day is as follows:

I am in the surgery shortly after 8 a.m., preparing for the treatment for the day. The first appointment is at 8.30. The day can be very varied from a straight forward filling to complicated bridge work, and I have to make sure that the dentist has everything he needs.

As well as mixing the materials for fillings and dental impressions, I assist with taking X rays, and reassuring patients. I still go to training courses to keep up to date with changes. I have been at this surgery for ten years now, so I know a lot of the patients and their families. The most enjoyable part of the job is that every day is different, and I feel I am really using my skills. We see everyone from young children, having their first check up, women who are expecting babies and older people.

The work can be quite tiring and I am pleased to put my feet up at the end of the day. It is nice having the weekends free.

NURSING IN HOSPITAL

Nursing posts in hospital can either be in surgical or medical settings, outpatients or in mental health care.

● CASE STUDY ● CASE STUDY ● CASE STUDY ● CASE STUDY ● CASE STUDY ● CASE STUDY ●

Sally is a staff nurse on a busy medical ward of 28 beds. Sally returned to nursing recently, having had two children. Once they were at secondary school, Sally decided she wanted to go back to nursing so she approached her local hospital who arranged for her to go on a retraining course for 12 weeks. During this time, Sally spent time on different wards and at the end of the retraining she was offered part time work. She works 4 days a week from 7.30 to 4 p.m. When she arrives on the ward in the morning, she receives the report from the night staff and uses the computer to log in the names of patients in the ward. Many records are now kept on computer, although patients

(continued)

also have written notes. During the day Sally gives out medicines, gives injections, changes dressings, talks to relatives, admits new patients, deals with emergency situations that could include coping with a patient whose heart stops beating and needs resuscitation.

Sally also teaches procedures to student nurses. At the moment the ward is divided into sections for men and women, and because of this layout there is a great deal of walking. Sally enjoys the pace of work and the variety of work – every day is different. The stresses of the job include being short staffed, never having enough time to spend time with patients and relatives and the endless paperwork.

Nursing team leader for Mental Health

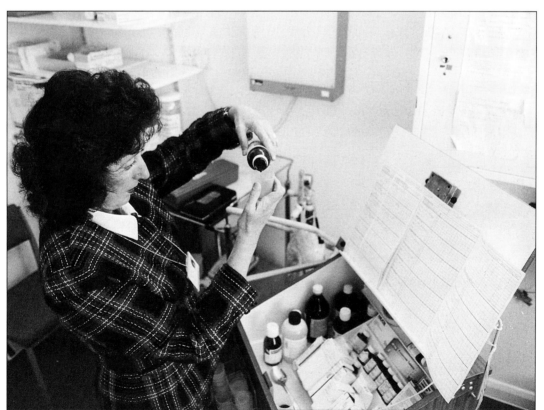

FIGURE 1.26 *Nursing team leader for Mental Health.*

● CASE STUDY ● CASE STUDY ● CASE STUDY ● CASE STUDY ● CASE STUDY ● CASE STUDY ●

Nursing team leader for Mental Health (continued)

Mary Andrews trained as a Registered Mental Nurse, and has specialised in Mental health in hospital ever since. She is responsible for a team of 23 nursing staff. The nurses are trained staff like Mary, and also NVQ nursing assistants. She is in charge of 181 mental health beds.

These include secure wards (which are kept locked), acute wards (where people may have tried to commit suicide) and long stay wards for people with dementia. Mary works 5 days a week, but is also on a rota for on-call duties at weekends and nights. She attends a lot of meetings with community nurses and voluntary organisations who are caring for people in the community with mental health problems. Mary is employed by the Hospital and Community Mental Health Trust. She enjoys her job and describes it as "challenging". Every day is different and she never knows what emergency she will deal with next. It can be stressful working with anxious relatives and also with people with violent or challenging behaviour, but Mary would not want to do anything else!

Jobs in Social Care

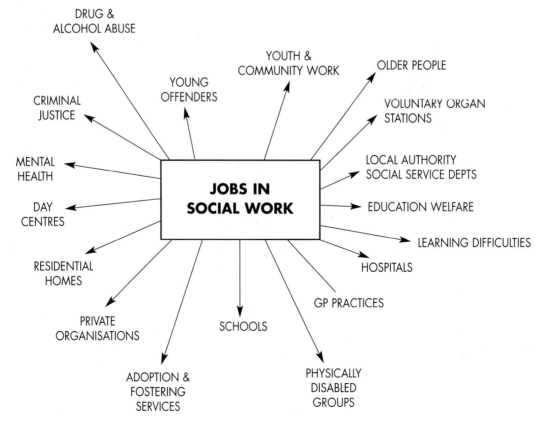

DIAGRAM 1.5 *The range of jobs in social work.*

Diagram 1.5 shows the range of jobs that are available in social work. At the moment qualified social workers have to take a 2 year Diploma course or a Degree in Social Work. The qualifications are currently being reviewed, and all qualifying programmes are likely to take 3 years in the future.

Most professional social workers are employed as "field" social workers. This means they work in the community or institution and have certain client groups. If you turn back to the diagram showing the structure of the typical Social Services department (fig 1.12), you can see that social workers are attached to a range of client groups, families and children, people with mental health problems, people with learning difficulties etc.

Social workers can be employed in private organisations or by voluntary groups. Social workers also work in hospitals, and this often involves liaising with other local council services for people returning home.

● CASE STUDY ● CASE STUDY ● CASE STUDY ● CASE STUDY ● CASE STUDY ● CASE STUDY ●

Debbie is a Social Worker, employed by a Social Services Department, in the Children and Families section. Debbie is responsible for following up incidents of non–accidental injury that have been reported by the local A and E department. Each day Debbie sees children and families and makes an assessment of their needs. She may provide them with advice, counselling or put them in touch with other agencies who may be able to help them, such as Child Psychiatry for family problems or Social Security for financial assistance. Although Debbie works 9 to 5, Monday to Friday, she is also on call some weekends and evenings. Apart from doing initial assessments, Debbie may help some families over a longer period of time with problems such as money, housing or relationship problems. She will attend regular case conferences for children who have been identified as "at risk" by Social Services. In these meetings she will discuss the family with the other professionals involved and make a Child Protection Plan to keep the children safe. The focus is on supporting and helping families care for their children properly. It is only in very exceptional circumstances when a child has suffered significant harm that she would apply to the Court to take the child into care. When she does this, she has to prove to the Court that the Social Services could do a better job than the family of looking after the child.

SOCIAL CARE

Social care workers can include people with NVQs (National Vocational Qualifications) and other qualifications and also unqualified people. They often work under the supervision of the social worker or qualified nurse.

Social care jobs are usually found in three main areas:

● domiciliary care (people being looked after in their own home)

● residential care

● day care

Figure 1.27 shows the job description for a home carer who will be looking after someone in their own home.

DEPARTMENT OF SOCIAL SERVICES

Post: Home carer

General purpose of job: to provide 7 day personal care and domestic help to people living in their own homes. Service users will be older people, families with children and people with a disability or mental illness, including those with carers such as relatives or friends. The post holder will be a team member committed to providing a caring service which puts the user first.

Personal care:

1 Assist with day to day grooming, washing, bathing and dressing, getting the user up and putting to bed

2 Help with toileting, dealing with incontinence and catheter care, emptying and disinfecting commodes

3 Assist with feeding, including preparation of meals and awareness of special dietary needs

4 Administration of medication prescribed by a doctor, including applying creams and inserting eye drops

Domestic care:

5 To undertake general housework, bed making and changing bed linen

6 Washing personal clothing and household in users home or local laundrette, or day centre by prior arrangement, ironing and mending

7 Shop, pay bills, collect pensions and prescriptions

8 Assist with financial affairs, keeping accurate records of all transactions

9 Help with correspondence and letter writing

10 Assist with pets

General duties

11 Write detailed reports on users progress and changes in their behaviour, needs or circumstances on a care plan in the users home. To notify the team leader of any such changes

12 Attend training sessions and meeting such as team meetings, case conferences and supervision sessions are required

13 Be responsible and handle emergencies with users in non-office hours which may require the carer to make a decision to call medical or emergency aid

14 Accompany the user to to pre-arranged appointments and occasional shopping trips, outings as required

15 Liaise with other professionals involved with the user e.g. GP, social worker, care manager, warden

16 Carers may hold keys for their users and must be responsible for their safe keeping

17 To establish a relationship with the user, give support to those under stress and provide companionship and a link with the community

18 Work in accordance with the department policies, practice and legislation relevant to their work, in particular operational, Health & Safety at work complaints

19 Must carry out all duties in accordance with the Council's equal opportunities policy

20 Any other comparable duties required by the line manager

FIGURE 1.27 *Job description of a home carer.*

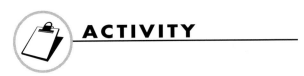

ACTIVITY

What skills are needed in this job? (refer to Diagram 1.4).

Compare the job description of the home carer with Figure 1.27 which is the job description for someone working in a residential home:

··

Day care assistant

Role:

1 To assist resident with their personal hygiene, grooming and with meals whenever necessary

2 To remember residents come first. Their care, well–being, personal comfort and happiness must be foremost in your mind at all times

Accountability:

The Care Assistant will take instruction from the Principal or Senior Care Assistant when carrying out duties

Duties:

1 Take report of previous shift with with Senior Care Assistant or Principal, note any changes in residents health and well–being, and in household routines

2 Clear all breakfast trays from rooms including water glasses and medicine pots before residents get up

3 Assist residents with dressing, washing and bathing where necessary

4 Assist with mobility problems e.g. to the lift, lavatory, dining room, etc

5 Make beds and remove hot water bottles, empty commodes, reporting any noticable changes in contents

6 Observe and report any changes in residents physical and emotional health

7 Prepare dining room for meals and serve them

8 Prepare residents for visits from doctors, district nurses, chiropodist, etc

9.1 Take over laundry duties in an emergency

9.2 Distribute clean laundry to residents

10 To assist with the administering of medication under the instruction of and in the presence of the senior person in charge

Other responsabilities:

1 To maintain a high standard of hygiene throughout the home

2 To perform duties with due regard to Health & Safety at Work procedures

3 To be fully aware of emergency procedures

4 To adapt to changing circumstances and techniques as they arise

5 To maintain a high standard of personal hygiene and grooming

6 To complete and sign a weekly time sheet

7 To report any defects in equipment and building to the principal immediately they are discovered

8 To have a cheerful and helpful approach to all visitors

Remember – the image of the home is greatly influenced by your attitude to them

FIGURE 1.28 *Day care assistant.*

Give examples from each job description of the following:

● Working as part of a team
● Working independently
● Being trustworthy
● Attention to hygiene
● Following instructions
● Communication skills
● Written skills

The job descriptions tend to focus on tasks that the worker has to do, but as we will see in the later section of this chapter, the care worker has to carry out these tasks taking account of the individual needs of the client.

CARING FOR CHILDREN

Workers in child care may have a range of qualifications. Diagram 1.6 shows the main jobs looking after children:

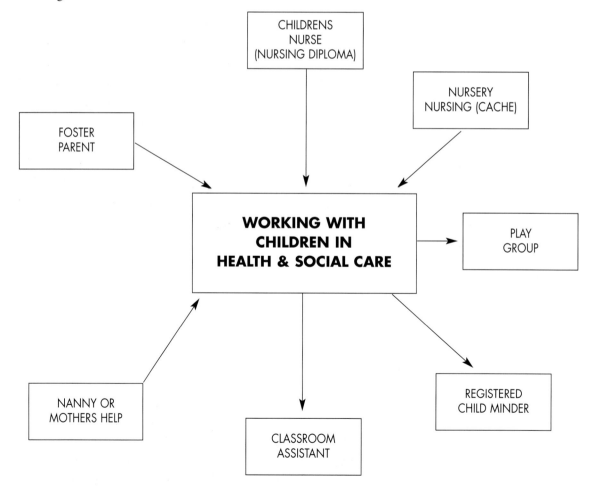

DIAGRAM 1.6 *Main jobs working with children in health and social care.*

Professions allied to Medicine (PAMS)

In addition to medicine and nursing, there are a number of roles within the health care occupational area. Examples of PAMS include the following:

➡ Speech Therapist
➡ Occupational Therapist
➡ Radiographer
➡ Radiotherapist

These qualifications all require a 3 year degree course at university, but there are also opportunities for people to work as assistants to these workers.

● CASE STUDY ● CASE STUDY ● CASE STUDY ● CASE STUDY ● CASE STUDY ● CASE STUDY ●

Helen completed her BTEC National Diploma in Health Studies, and gained a degree in physiotherapy. She is working in a busy physio department in a Hospital Trust. On a typical day, Helen can spend most of the morning visiting the wards and assisting people with breathing exercises and other exercises after operations or illnesses. She spends quite a lot of time on the medical ward encouraging people who have had a stroke to improve their mobility and the use of their affected limbs. In the afternoon, she works in the department with a range of people who have been referred by their GPs or Hospital consultants. Treatment can include the use of heat, applying traction, massage and ultrasound treatment, as well as advising patients on appropriate exercises. Some heart patients need to improve their circulation with work in the gym, including exercise bikes and the treadmill. Helen really wants to specialise in sports injuries. Many of the patients she sees have been referred because of injuries, and with more people taking up sport and other activities Helen thinks this area of work will increase in the future.

So far in this section, we have looked at jobs that give direct care to patients in the community and in the hospital, but there are several workers in GP practices who give support to doctors and nurses.

Administration staff

Practice managers

These are key people in the practice, in charge of the receptionists, secretaries and other workers. They have overall responsibility for the smooth running of the surgeries. Responsibilities include making sure that the computers are working and making appointments for drug representatives to see the doctors. They make sure that all staff working in the practice are aware of health and safety issues. They interview new staff and provide an induction to the practice. They are responsible for the holiday rota system, and they deal with complaints from patients.

Practice managers have a wide range of backgrounds. They could have previous experience in social care or nursing, but they have to have good office skills. In order to become a practice manager, you have to take the Diploma in Practice Management.

Receptionist

Receptionists are the first person the patient comes into contact with when entering the surgery or when phoning with a query or to make an appointment. Many patients are very anxious when they call on the receptionist. The receptionist must be careful to be aware of issues of confidentiality. If a patient telephones the surgery wanting to know the result of a test, there are usually clear guidelines about the correct procedure to be followed, and the doctor will usually speak to the patient personally if there is an abnormal result. Receptionists may hear details of a private nature being discussed, and it is very important that these matters are not referred to elsewhere.

Figure 1.29 shows the organisation of a health centre:

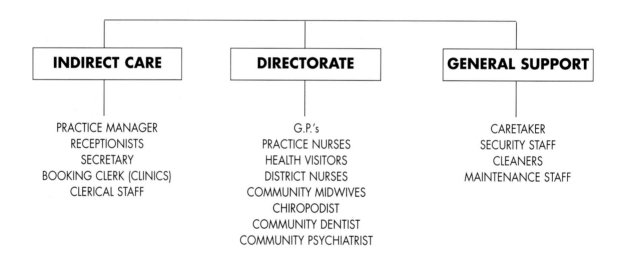

FIGURE 1.29 *Diagram of a health centre.*

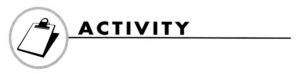

ACTIVITY

We have now looked at several examples of jobs in the hospital and in the community. Are the same qualities required for each job, or are they different? Look again at the list of qualities in diagram 1.4 and think what qualities are needed for each of the jobs we have discussed in this section.

Early Years Services

There is an overlap in services provided for the health care, social care and education services provided for children.

Primary Health Care

Most care of young children is undertaken by parents. With less time spent in hospital, children are more likely to be looked after in their own homes. GPs have responsibility for all the children in their practice. Preventative services such as routine immunisations, developmental checks and advising parents are all part of the work of the Primary Health Care Team (PHCT).

DISEASE	TIME	COMMON REACTIONS	PROTECTION
Diphtheria, whooping cough (Pertussis), tetanus (also known as DTP or triple vaccine)	Injections at 2, 3, and 4 months; repeat diphtheria + tetanus at $3\frac{1}{2}$–5 years	Child may become feverish; the site of the injection may be sore	Repeat at school leaving age
Polio	Oral vaccine at 2, 3 and 4 months; repeat at $3\frac{1}{2}$–5 years	None	Repeat at school leaving age and every 10 years, if travelling to high risk countries
MMR – measles, mumps, German measles (rubella)	Injection at 12–15 months; repeated at $3\frac{1}{2}$–5 years or earlier	Child may become feverish and have a slight rash for 7–10 days after vaccination	Further doses are not recommended after 2 injections
Tuberculosis (BCG)	Injection at 10–13 years to all school children not immune	The site of the injection may be sore and stiff	Unknown
Hib (Haemophilus influenza Hib type B) Hib meningitis, epiglottis, septicaemia, septic arthritis, osteomyelitis, pneumonia	Injection at 2, 3 and 4 months, or just one injection for children over a year old	The site of the injection may become red and swollen	After 4 years of age the child should have developed a natural resistance to Hib and does not need to be immunised
Meningococcal C, meningitis, septicaemia	As Hib above	As Hib above	Long lasting. A booster not currently recommended

FIGURE 1.30 *Immunisation table: Health Authority immunisation schedule.*

Figure 1.30 is an immunisation table that shows the times at which children will have their jabs.

School services

The Government's Healthier Schools Programme means healthier children. School nurses promote the health of the children and give help and advice to parents and pupils. Each school has a named doctor and nurse who visit the school regularly and refer children to other services in the community.

THE PAEDIATRIC COMMUNITY TEAM

JOB/TITLE	SERVICES & SUPPORT FOR:	REFERRAL BY
Health visitor	Infant feeding and nutrition, Child development, behavioural problems	GP, midwife, self referral
Audiology service	Children who have hearing problems or are behind with language development	Health visitor, school nurse, GP, self referral
Speech and language therapist	Children who stammer, children under 6 who cannot pronounce words properly, young babies and children who have difficulty eating and drinking	GP, health visitor, school nurse
Community paediatrician	Minor and major health problems in babies and young children, children with special needs, developmental problems	GP, heal;th visitor, school nurse
Child and adolescent psychiatrist or family therapist	Depression, eating disorders, disruptive behaviour, bereavement problems, abuse, self abuse	GP, health visitor, school nurse teacher
Educational and clinical psychologist	Family crisis, bullying, anxiety, problems at school	Educational authority, school nurse, teacher
Sleep and behaviour clinics (run by health visitor or/and psychiatrist	Sleep problems, toddler tantrums, toileting problems, aggression	GP, health visitor, school nurse
Community dental service (dentist)	Pre-school or school child with special needs who need dental care at home	Dentist, GP
Enuresis clinic (bedwetting service) (run by health visitor)	Bedwetting in children and teenagers	School nurse, health visitor, GP

TABLE 1.4 *The paediatric community team.*

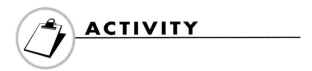

ACTIVITY

Table 1.4 shows the children services available in the community. After you have studied it, look at the following case studies and decide which service should be used for each child (you could refer to more than one service if you think it is necessary). (See end of Chapter for Answers.)

1 Jason, aged 3, is very jealous of his baby sister. He keeps biting and pinching her. He also very aggressive in the nursery classroom.

2 Bella, aged 4, has cerebral palsy and has difficulty swallowing.

3 Shakira is 6 and still wets the bed at night. She finds it embarrassing as she wants to stay overnight at her friends' house.

4 David, aged 6, has learning difficulties. It is impossible for his mother to take him to the dentist in the High Street. She has noticed that his teeth are stained and dirty, and she has difficulty teaching David how to clean his teeth.

5 Jane has just had twins. She is trying to breast feed them without success.

6 Rosie, who is 4, has had continuous ear infections for the last year, and ignores her mother when she calls her in from the garden.

7 Anna is 14 months old and cannot sit up on her own yet. She seems to have problems seeing things, her mother thinks she has a squint.

8 Maria is 8 and wants to be a model when she grows up. Her mother has discovered that she has not been eating her packed lunch at school. When she changes for games the teacher notices she has scratches and cuts on her arms.

9 Rania is 7. Her parents divorced recently and she is living with her mother. She is very disruptive in class. She will not sit down, but runs round the classroom, shouting and causing a disturbance.

Apart from these community services, there are also paediatric nurses employed by the Hospital or Community Trusts who visit children in their own homes to continue treatment or to offer support after a stay in hospital. The duties of a community paediatric nurse can include the following:

➡ follow up care after treatment in A and E

➡ post operative care

➡ removal of stitches, dressing of wounds, giving injections

➡ advising and training parents in giving care

EMERGENCY MEDICAL SERVICES FOR CHILDREN

Apart from the out of hours service offered by GPs, there are specialist children's hospitals that look after children until the age of 16. The hospital is organised so that children feel comfortable. Often the departments and wards are brightly painted with pictures and other decorations.

Secondary Health Services for Early Years

Secondary care is provided in hospitals. Hospital paediatricians provide emergency and routine surgery for children. GPs will refer children to Outpatient Departments where children can be seen by the specialist team. Nowadays parents are encouraged to stay with their children in hospital and overnight accommodation is offered to them.

Hospital Play Specialist

A Hospital play specialist is usually a trained nursery nurse who has additional training in supporting children through play. Operations and procedures can be explained to the child using dolls. Play is also used to relieve stress

Social Services Early Years

The local social service departments provide a range of services to young children. These services may be provided directly by social services, provided in partnership with voluntary organisations or they are purchased from private or other independent sector providers.

Statutory provision

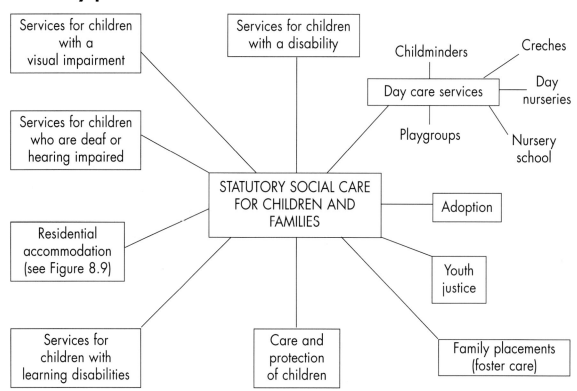

FIGURE 1.31 *A summary for statutory social care for children and families.*

Thomas & Meggitt, Human Growth and Development, Hodder & Stoughton

Figure 1.31 shows the services that must be provided by the Social Services. The Children Act (1989) was an important piece of legislation that stated the follow up services must be provided for those children assessed as being in need.

1 day care for children under 5 and not at school

2 care and supervised activities outside school hours and during school holidays

3 accommodation if required, if children are lost, abandoned or without a carer that can provide accommodation.

They must also provide:

➡ assessment of needs

➡ an emergency service 24 hours a day, 365 days a year

Social Services may also provide the following caring services for children and their families:

➡ occupational therapy

➡ supplying specialist equipment

➡ respite care

➡ personal help

Day care Services and Childminders

Childminders must be registered with the local authority, and they are inspected and registered annually.

FOSTERING AND ADOPTION

The Children Act (1989) states that the Local Authority must make arrangements to enable the child to live with their families unless this would harm the child. Foster carers are approved by either the local authority or by a voluntary or private organisation. Local Authorities have to keep a register of foster carers in the area and keep records of children placed with them.

The law related to Adoption is complicated (Adoption Act 1979 and Children Act 1989). An adoption order transfers all the responsibilities of the parent to the adopters.

An adopter has to be:

● at least 21

● resident in the UK

● able to meet the criteria of the relevant adoption agency or local authority

RESIDENTIAL CARE FOR EARLY YEARS

Figure 1.32 summarises the residential accommodation for Early Years for which the local authority has responsibility. At the moment the Inspection unit of the local authority inspects residential homes twice a year. One of these visits is announced, which means that the home has notice when to expect a visit. The other visit is unannounced, when the home does not receive notice when the inspector arrives. Why do you think it is important to have unannounced inspections?

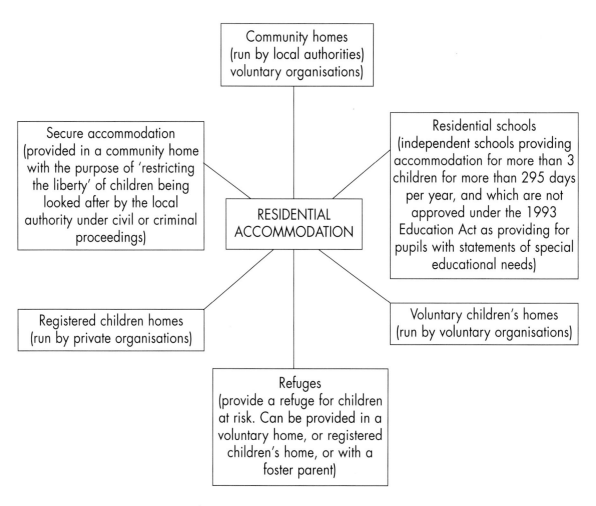

FIGURE 1.32 *Residential accommodation for children*

There has been a great deal of concern about the level of abuse in Children's Homes; the Inspection procedures are now being reviewed. As well as trained full time inspectors, lay people who have been trained as "lay assessors" will accompany the inspectors on their visits.

In the future the Inspection Unit will become separate from the Local Authority. Why do you think it is important to have unannounced inspections?

NON-STATUTORY PROVISION

Local Authorities provide some non-statutory provision, such as training for childminders.

Other examples of non-statutory provision would include:

- private nurseries
- private residential homes
- private fostering and adoption agencies

These are privately run as businesses, but the providers have to be registered and inspected by the local authority.

Independent voluntary provision for Early Years can include:

➡ toddlers clubs

➡ care for children with Special Needs (e.g. Mencap services)

➡ holiday care

➡ mother and child support groups

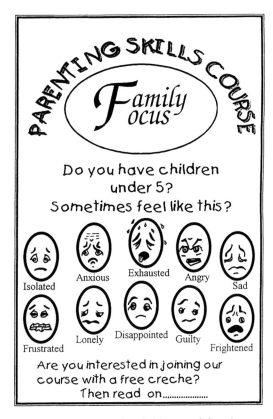

FIGURE 1.33 *Example of a voluntary service for children and families.*

Figure 1.33 is an example of a voluntary service for mothers with young children. Family Focus is a registered charity which was set up protect and preserve the mental and physical health of families with children under 5. Family Focus aims to:

➡ work alongside parents to develop family life skills

➡ to help parents enjoy parenthood

➡ to help parents cope with the daily pressures of life

To do this, parents can take part in a parenting skills course which includes:

➡ child development

➡ managing behaviour

➡ meeting needs of children and parents

➡ the importance of play

There are also other charities involved with the protection of young children. The most well known of these is the NSPCC (National Society for the Prevention of Cruelty to Children). The NSPCC advises parents on child care, supports families who are finding it difficult to cope with their children as well as investigating cases of abuse and cruelty to children.

Informal provision

Much of the care of young children is arranged on an informal basis. For example, friends and neighbours may do unpaid babysitting; local churches may run mother and toddler clubs.

EFFECTIVE COMMUNICATION SKILLS

The health and social care worker must be able to communicate effectively with a wide range of patients or clients:

- babies/children
- adolescents
- young adults
- older people
- other health workers
- doctors
- nurses
- teachers
- police
- social workers

Lack of effective communication between the care worker and the patient will mean that the client will not receive the support they need.

Communication can take many forms. We will look at alternative forms of communication for people with specific problems later in the chapter. In this section we will be looking at communication in the form of:

➡ verbal communication

➡ non-verbal communication

➡ written communication

VERBAL COMMUNICATION

Everyone says they know how to talk, but in health and social care it is important to use verbal communication effectively:

➡ in assessing patients

➡ identifying needs

➡ giving information

➡ encouraging patients to express their own views and be independent

Questions

Most health and social workers use questions every day. There are several types of question:

Closed Questions

For example 'How old are you?'
'What is your name?'
'Are you married?'

These questions are appropriate when brief factual material is needed, but they do not encourage conversation and expression of thoughts and feelings.

Open (or Open ended) Questions

These give an opportunity for fuller deeper answers:

e.g. 'How do you feel about moving into sheltered housing?'
'Is there anything you need to know about how to breast feed the baby?'

How, **what**, **feel** and **think** are useful words for encouraging a full response.

Biased Questions

These indicate the answer the questioner wants or expects to hear:

e.g. 'You have settled into the routine of the home, haven't you?'
'It isn't necessary to go over your medication again, is it?'

Multiple questions

These include more than one question and can cause confusion"
e.g. 'Is this a serious problem, when did it start?'
'How did the accident happen, what did you do?'

It is the responsibility of the health and social care worker to make sure that communication is effective.

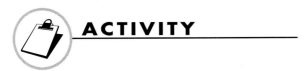 **ACTIVITY**

Which of the following questions are closed, open, biased, or multiple? (See end of Chapter for Answers.)

1 How are you?
2 How often do you come to the surgery?
3 Have you collected your repeat prescriptions, which ones do you have?
4 You prefer to do your own shopping don't you?

Communication is a two way process:

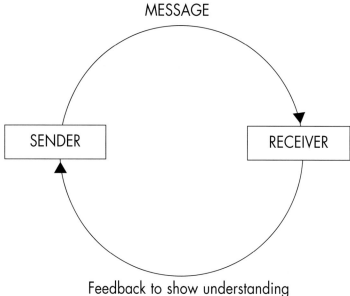

DIAGRAM 1.7 *The circle of communication*

Diagram 1.7 shows the circle of communication.

The sender is the care worker; the receiver is the patient who hears, sees or reads the message. In order for communication to take place the receiver has to understand the message, and give feedback to the sender that the message has been understood.

We all communicate every day. Think about a typical day in your life and the communications that take place.

You may have identified some of the following:

➡ informal conversation with friends, either one to one or else in a group

➡ more formal discussions at work or college

➡ telephone conversations, formal and informal

➡ letters from friends, emails, faxes

All these forms of communication use words, either spoken or written. Think about a recent communication that went well. Why did it go well? Now think about a recent communication that left you feeling awkward, angry, or frustrated. What was the problem?

Barriers to communication can include the following:

● Insufficient information is given

● The environment is unhelpful, noisy, lack of privacy, too many people talking at the same time

● The other person does not seem interested to hear what you have to say

● Lack of understanding due to language used

Can you think of why you had problems in a recent communication?

Listening skills

Listening skills are very important in health and social care. In ordinary conversations there tends to be a pattern to conversation. For example: Mary tells Surinder about what she did on Saturday night, and Surinder tells Mary what she did on Saturday night. We can see that there is an exchange of information. In effective listening the pattern is different. In effective listening you need to concentrate on the feelings of the other person and put your own views and feelings to one side.

Look at the following conversation:

Mrs Hill: *"Ever since my husband died last year, I have felt very lonely and depressed, and it is a real effort to do anything."*

Care worker: *"Oh, I know how you feel. When my husband died I felt dreadful for ages, and I still miss him now."*

What is the problem with the care workers response?

You can see that the care worker is more concerned with expressing her own feelings, rather than listening effectively to Mrs Hill.

Listening effectively can be developed through the method called "reflecting back". The care worker checks that they are fully understanding what the client is saying, by restating what has been said. This helps the client to make their feeling clear. Reflecting back is used in the discussion of feelings, not in other situations.

Read this example of reflecting back:

Mother: *"I just feel so useless. I never realised having a baby was such hard work. I seem to run about all day and I never get the place straight, and I feel so tired."*

Health Visitor: *"Why do you think you feel so tired?*

Mother: *"I suppose I feel I want everything to be perfect. My mother-in -law lives nearby. She is always popping in. Her house always looks perfect. She must think I am useless."*

Health Visitor: *"Why do you think your mother-in-law thinks you are useless?"*

Mother: *"She has never approved of me, and it is even worse now."*

Health Visitor: *"You think it has got worse since you had the baby?"*

By reflecting back in this way, the health worker may be able to help the patient identify the real problem. In this case, the problem may be the relationship between the two women, rather than the birth of the new baby. On the other hand, it could be that the mother has post–natal depression. In either case, effective listening is a useful tool in helping people to understand their feelings.

Reflecting back is a skill but needs to be used appropriately. We have seen programmes about social workers whose catch phrase is "I hear what you are saying". This can be irritating to the client. Catch phrases are not enough, you need to practise listening skills.

 ACTIVITY

1   **Working with a partner, move your chairs so you are sitting back to back. Without turning round, take it in turns to talk to each other, one acting as speaker, the other acting as listener. The one acting as listener is not allowed to say anything, and that includes grunting, laughing.**

    When you have finished, discuss how you felt, as a listener, and as a talker.

2   **Sitting face to face, take it in turns to act as listener and talker. This time the listener avoids looking at the speaker during their conversation.**

    How does this feel?

    From these exercises we can see that communication skills do not just include listening and talking, but they also include non–verbal communication.

NON–VERBAL COMMUNICATION

Non–verbal communication is communication without words. The following are examples of non-verbal communication:

➡ physical contact – touching, holding hands, hugging etc
➡ proximity – how close you sit or stand when you are talking to people
➡ posture – how you stand or sit, crossed arms, crossed legs, leaning forward
➡ gestures – what you do with your hands and arms, also nodding or shaking your head
➡ facial expression – smiling, laughing, frowning
➡ eye contact and movement – staring, blinking, winking, looking at someone
➡ tone of voice – loud, soft, aggressive
➡ pace of voice – speaking fast, slow, hesitating

The reasons why you found the first exercise uncomfortable is that we look at the person we are talking to in order to gain a response, and we can respond using non–verbal communication as well to reinforce the communication process. The second exercise also demonstrates the importance of eye contact when communicating with someone.

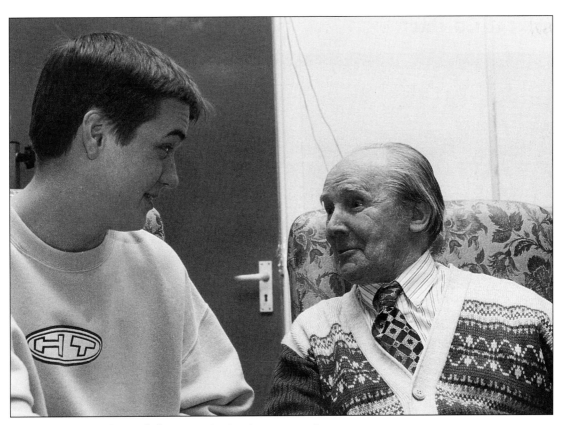

FIGURE 1.34 *Non verbal communication in a care setting.*

Look at Figure 1.34. This is a photograph of Philip, a volunteer worker talking to a client at a day centre. Make a list of non–verbal communication you can see.

Philip is looking at Mr Tate, he is smiling and he is sitting in his chair at the same level at Mr Tate. Another interesting thing we can see here, is that Philip is reflecting Mr Tate's facial expression; look at the raised eyebrows in both men. This is called mirroring, and is often done unconsciously when people are trying to establish an equal relationship.

Next time you are in a bar, or in the college dining room, make a note of the non–verbal communication you can see occurring between two people. Not only may you see facial expressions mirrored, but you may see other gestures reflected by the couples, such as touching their own hair, hand movements etc. We need to be aware of non–verbal communication, and also how some forms of verbal communication may be appropriate in some situations and not in others.

PHYSICAL CONTACT

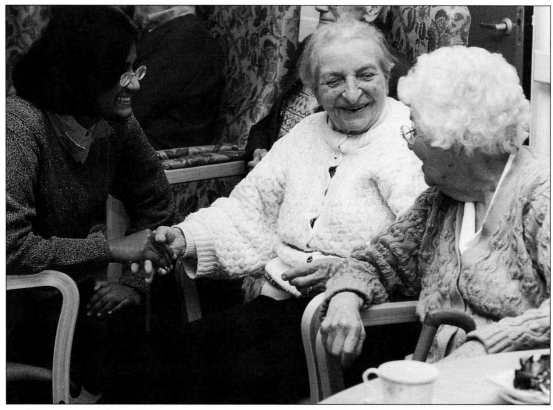

FIGURE 1.35 *Using interpersonal skills.*

Health and social care workers often touch patients and clients in order to show support and understanding. Look at figure 1.35. The photograph shows Ashna, a volunteer at a day centre, with two of the clients. Note the non–verbal communication that is shown by all the people in the photograph. You can see that Ashna is holding Mrs Gibson's hand. Why do you think she is doing this? Would you think it was appropriate if Ashna was a male carer? As care workers we need to be aware of the appropriate use of touch, especially on different parts of the body. The hands and arms are usually seen as acceptable areas to touch, but to touch other parts of the body, such as thigh, neck or knee would be seen as off limits unless you are massaging or washing someone. Again, there are cultural differences. Asian women would not wish to be touched by a man. Because of problems of accusations of abuse, all care workers need to be aware of the appropriate use of touch.

Look at these statements and decide which ones are true and which ones are false. (See end of Chapter for Answers.)

1   People are more likely to talk to those with whom they feel safe.
2   People who can't wait to say something themselves are good at listening.
3   People who are tired or stressed find it difficult to listen to others.
4   Talking is more important than listening.
5   People who feel very emotional about issues make good listeners.
6   Talking to patients is time wasted; you should be doing useful work instead.

7   It is hard to be a good listener.

8   Patients may find it difficult to talk about personal issues.

We have discussed communication; now it is your turn to practise your own communication skills. **Working in groups or pairs try the following role plays:**

1   You are the receptionist in a busy GP Practice. Mrs Hall telephones you and demands an immediate appointment with the doctor. Mrs Hall starts the conversation by saying:

"I really must see the doctor today" in an aggressive tone of voice. How do you deal with this?

2   You are the clinic clerk in hospital, booking in patients for future appointments. You are on duty on your own today. A long queue is forming and people are beginning to look at their watches and complain to each other. How do you use verbal and non–verbal communication in this situation?

3   Working on the maternity unit, you answer the phone. A male voice asks how Charlotte Spencer is. Charlotte is a teenager who is having a difficult pregnancy and her mother is her next of kin. How do you respond to the caller? (be careful of confidentiality).

4   You are a care worker in a residential home. You know Mr Patel is a diabetic and you see him eating some chocolates that have been given to the home. What do you say?

5   You are an occupational therapist making a home assessment on Mrs Khan's mobility in her home. You need to assess how well she will cope at home after a recent operation. You notice frayed carpets and trailing flexes in the living room that may cause an accident. How do you start the conversation with her daughter?

6   You are a dental nurse and as part of your role you have to advise patients on how to clean their teeth properly. How might you change your approach for:

➡   a young child

➡   a teenager

➡   an older man

➡   a pregnant woman

Discussion

As you can see in all 6 cases, it isn't just the words you say that are important, but the tone of voice, posture, facial expression, and gestures. On the phone, the tone of voice is very important, and you also have to speak more clearly and slowly as the person you are speaking to cannot see you for additional non verbal information. If you become impatient or aggressive with an aggressive patient or client, the situation can get worse, so it is important to keep calm before you say anything.

Useful Strategies

1   If something isn't clear, ask for additional information. Sometimes this slows down the communication and can reduce tension.

2   Take a deep breath and speak slowly and clearly.

3   Maintain eye contact if face to face, and try to sit down rather than stand up, as people are more relaxed if they are sitting down. If the patient is in bed or in a chair make sure you are at the same level, rather than standing over them.

4   Respect issues of confidentiality.

5   Don't try to score points or put people down.

THE BENEFITS OF EFFECTIVE COMMUNICATION

For the care worker

- can obtain and provide useful information that is relevant to client's/patient's well–being
- enables care worker to support and understand the client/patient
- assists team work
- can help patients make their needs known

If communication is not effective:

- patients can feel angry and resentful
- patients feel they are not being listened to and understood
- patients don't understand why certain procedures are happening
- patients may not follow treatment and exercise that may help them recover

We will be looking at certain groups with specific communication problems in the next section.

WRITTEN COMMUNICATION

In Health and Social Care work, written communication is very important.

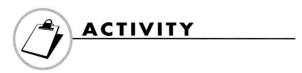 **ACTIVITY**

Make a list of written communication used in health and social care.

Your list could include:

- **patient records**
- **care plans**
- **referral letters**
- **accident report forms**
- **prescriptions**
- **consent forms**

Patients' records are legal documents and could be used in a court of law. It is important they are:

- clear
- can be read easily
- concise
- based on fact and not on opinion

Consider these 2 examples of a patient record of Mrs Brown who is on the medical ward:

Example A

Mrs Brown had a good night.

Example B

Mrs Brown slept for 6 hours without medication. She woke up at 6 a.m. and said she was free from pain, and did not require a pain killer.

Discussion

In Example A. "a good night," could mean anything. It is vague and does not give any information.

In Example B. We know that Mrs Brown slept for 6 hours, she was not in pain, and did not need a painkiller. The use of Mrs Brown's own words is also seen as a reliable record.

OTHER FORMS OF COMMUNICATION

MONDAY	☺ HOORAY	☺ 50/50	☹ OOPS !	MONDAY	☺ HOORAY	☺ 50/50	☹ OOPS !
TUESDAY	☺ GREAT	☺ 50/50	☹ OH DEAR !	TUESDAY	☺ GREAT	☺ 50/50	☹ OH DEAR !
WEDNESDAY	☺ BRILLIANT	☺ 50/50	☹ NEVER MIND	WEDNESDAY	☺ BRILLIANT	☺ 50/50	☹ NEVER MIND
THURSDAY	☺ YES	☺ 50/50	☹ TRY AGAIN	THURSDAY	☺ YES	☺ 50/50	☹ TRY AGAIN
FRIDAY	☺ O.K. MAN	☺ 50/50	☹ WHOOPSY	FRIDAY	☺ O.K. MAN	☺ 50/50	☹ WHOOPSY
SATURDAY	☺ GOOD	☺ 50/50	☹ GOOD LUCK	SATURDAY	☺ GOOD	☺ 50/50	☹ GOOD LUCK
SUNDAY	☺ FUNKY	☺ 50/50	☹ HARD LUCK	SUNDAY	☺ FUNKY	☺ 50/50	☹ HARD LUCK

MADE BY THOMAS MICHAEL GARROD©

FIGURE 1.36 *A child-friendly chart.*

Other forms of communication used in health and social care can include:

- posters (often to do with health promotion)
- leaflets
- diagrams

When communicating with children, leaflets may be too complicated, and diagrams may be more appropriate.

Figure 1.36 is an example of a record kept by a child who is attending an enuresis clinic (for bedwetting). NB It is clear and gives an encouraging message to the child. It is also easy for the nurse to check the progress that is being made. The child colours in the appropriate box.

PRINCIPLES OF GOOD PRACTICE AND THE CARE VALUE BASE

The Care Value Base underpins the work of everyone in health, social care and Early Years Services. The value base underpins all training in care. It is used as the basis for NVQs (National Vocational Qualifications) in acute care in hospitals, and care in residential homes, nurseries and domiciliary work.

The 5 Elements in the Value Base are as follows:

1 Promoting anti–discriminatory practice
2 Maintaining confidentiality of information
3 Promoting individuals' rights to dignity, independence and safety
4 Acknowledging individuals' personal beliefs and identity
5 Supporting individuals through effective communication

PROMOTING ANTI-DISCRIMINATORY PRACTICE

Discrimination occurs very frequently. Discrimination means that certain people are treated less favourably than others because of a personal characteristic they have.

Certain groups are more likely to experience discrimination. These are:

- people with learning difficulties
- older people
- people with physical disabilities
- people with mental health problems
- women
- minority ethnic groups
- minority religious groups
- gay men and lesbians

Discrimination may be direct or indirect

An example of direct discrimination would be a clear statement of different treatment for a certain group. Direct discrimination of certain groups is banned by law

The main Acts of Parliament that are relevant are:

The Race Relations Act (1976)

This Act bans all forms of racial discrimination in work, housing and the provision of services. The Act is being revised, to include indirect discrimination.

The Sex Discrimination Act (1975)

This Act provides equal rights to men and women in work, services and access to facilities. The Act covers both Direct and Indirect Discrimination.

Disability Discrimination Act (1995)

This Act gives rights to disabled people in employment, access to education and transport, housing and obtaining goods and services. However although the legislation exists there are examples where indirect discrimination occurs.

Word check
Direct Discrimination

A landlord puts a notice in the window for a lodger and says "No Irish or Blacks". You can see that this is a clear example of **direct** discrimination, with certain groups being treated unfairly. To write a notice like this would be illegal nowadays.

Indirect discrimination

What do you think of this advertisement?

Cook wanted for nursing home. Must be strong, be 6 foot tall and have a good standard of English, preferably GCSE at A to C. You could say that this is an example of indirect discrimination, because although the advert doesn't clearly state that it wants white males, the personal factors required make this likely. Not many women are 6 foot tall, and workers who have English as a second language are less likely to have GCSE at the standard stated.

If the advertiser was challenged over this advert, he /she would need to prove that the height and English qualification was an essential requirement of the job. At the moment age discrimination is not covered by legislation.

Look at this extract from the future prescribing plan from a health authority:

"It is not expected that prescriptions for this drug will be given to people over 75" This would appear to be an example of discrimination on the basis of age. The organisation Age Concern has collected evidence that older people may not be offered treatment and services because of their age (See Figure 1.37).

Ageist health barriers

Restore clinical need as the NHS gateway

Earlier this year a gallup poll of 1,600 people over 50 felt that they had been refused treatment on the grounds of their age – and 1 in 10 (almost 2m people if extrapolated nationwide) felt they had been treated differently since hitting 50. Age Concern, the pressure group which commissioned the April survey appealed to the public and health professionals for more evidence about age discrimination in the health service. Over 1,000 people responded. Today's report based on a close analysis of 150 cases, portrays a stark picture of systematic ageism within the NHS. It sets out the barriers which people over 50 face obtaining treatment, the less caring attitudes of health staff, and the way the fear of retaliation restricts complaints.

FIGURE 1.37 *Ageism.*

Other examples of discriminatory practice in health and social care could include the following:

➡ A nurse who applies for promotion but is rejected because she is taking drugs to control her epilepsy

➡ A nursery refuses to take a child with HIV

➡ A nursery who refuses to take a child who has a facial disfigurement, saying it will frighten the other children

➡ A teenager with Downs Syndrome who cannot find a dentist willing to take him on his list

➡ A refugee who cannot find a GP to take him on as a patient

People are treated unfairly because of prejudice and the use of stereotypes that are often reinforced by the media.

Prejudice is an attitude that develops towards a particular group that has been identified in a negative way. **Stereotypes** develop from a simplified image of a group.

For example

The **stereotype** of older people is that they are all deaf and act like children.

This can be reinforced through television and the media, so that unless you have personal experience of older people, when you care for an older person you may shout at them (thinking they are deaf) and suggest childish activities for them to do such as playing musical chairs.

Discrimination may be unconsciously done, but as care workers we must be careful not to use stereotypes when supporting patients and clients. At the same time, we need to be aware that everyone is an individual and we are not effective care workers if we treat everyone the same.

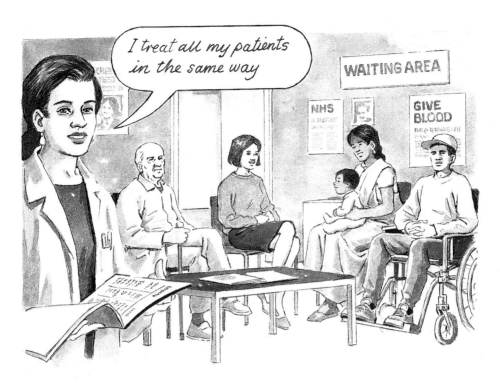

FIGURE 1.38 *Should all patients be treated the same way?*

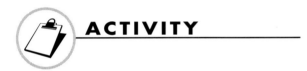ACTIVITY

Look at Figure 1.38 where the practice nurse is saying she treats everyone the same. What is the problem here? (See end of Chapter for Answers.)

. . . .

Discriminatory behaviour can include:

- racist and sexist jokes
- isolating clients with a mental health problem
- avoiding looking after someone who is from a different ethnic background from your own
- ignoring the needs of someone with HIV
- excluding certain residents from activities

Discriminatory behaviour can also be indicated through:

- tone of voice (loud and aggressive)
- body language (distant and threatening)
- eye gaze (avoiding eye contact, or glaring)

Most health and social care organisations have an equal opportunities policy. If you go on work experience try to look at the equal opportunities policy at the placement.

Although it is important to respect the values of clients and patients, you also need to be aware of the rights of other clients and service users and also safety issues.

● **CASE STUDY** ● **CASE STUDY** ● **CASE STUDY** ● **CASE STUDY** ● **CASE STUDY** ● **CASE STUDY** ●

John has learning difficulties and lives in a hostel with nine other men in their twenties, who also have learning difficulties. There is a smoking policy in the house. Smoking is allowed in one area downstairs. John says he wants to smoke upstairs in his room. The staff are concerned about the fire risk as two months earlier, John went to sleep with a lighted cigarette in his mouth, but the care assistant discovered him before any damage was done. John feels he is being treated unfairly because he has a learning disability.

● **CASE STUDY** ● **CASE STUDY** ● **CASE STUDY** ● **CASE STUDY** ● **CASE STUDY** ● **CASE STUDY** ●

In a residential home in East London, all the residents are white men and women in their seventies. The care assistants include Maria, who is Afro Caribbean. Mrs Bryant says "I don't want a darkie looking after me".

What should the home manager do in these situations?

In order to promote anti–discriminatory practice, health and care organisations should:

● develop policies
● implement them
● give staff training in promoting better care to all clients
● have a complaints procedure so that patients and clients can seek redress

All care workers find they like some of their patients more than others. This is natural. What you need to ask yourself is why you do not like a client? If it is because you feel awkward dealing with them because you do not understand their religion or culture, finding out about their views may be beneficial.

MAINTAINING THE CONFIDENTIALITY OF INFORMATION

Confidentiality is about keeping information private when it should be kept private. Think about the last time you went to see your doctor or practice nurse.

● What information would you be happy to give?
● What information would you feel uncomfortable about giving?

● How would you feel if your personal details were freely available to everyone?

A health and social care worker will know a great deal about the person they are looking after. It is essential that the information is kept confidential and not passed on without the clients' permission.

Some information may have to be passed on from one care worker to another, from a nurse to a doctor, but this must be done with the patient's permission. The death of a patient does not give you the right to break confidentiality.

Clause 10 of the Code of Professional Conduct for nurses states that:

"As a registered nurse, midwife or health visitor, you are personally accountable for your practice, and you must… protect all confidential information about patients and clients obtained in the course of professional practice and make disclosures only with consent, where required by the order of a court or where you can justify disclosure in the wider public interest" (UKCC).

Confidentiality can only be broken in exceptional circumstances. Patients and clients have a right to know that their personal details are kept private and confidential. If you, as the care worker, need to disclose information this should be done:

● with the consent of the client or patient – without the consent of the client or patient if required by law

● without the consent of the client or patient if the disclosure is seen to be in the public interest

● CASE STUDY ● CASE STUDY ● CASE STUDY ● CASE STUDY ● CASE STUDY ● CASE STUDY ●

You are working on a male medical ward. A young man is brought in as an emergency. He has a bag with him that he asks you to keep in a safe place. He tells you that he has just arrived from India, and he is taking Schedule A drugs to his brother. He asks you to keep his secret.

● CASE STUDY ● CASE STUDY ● CASE STUDY ● CASE STUDY ● CASE STUDY ● CASE STUDY ●

You are on night duty on the children's ward. One of the children tells you her stepfather is abusing her.

In both these cases the duty of the nurse is quite clear, as in both cases it is a matter of public interest, but a lot of cases are quite difficult, and you would need to discuss the case with your manager. In the 2 cases outlined above, you would first report the matter to your line manager.

Written Records

Medical records are also covered by the same principles of confidentiality. There are usually procedures for keeping records safe, in locked filing cabinets.

The 1987 Access to Personal Files Act meant that patients can see their personal medical or social service files from this date. Notice to view your records is required. Doctors charge a fee for this service, and any record that may be damaging to the patient (in the opinion of the doctor) can be with held. People with mental health problems could come into this category.

Sometimes patient's records need to be transferred if the patient is moving to another home, or if they have an appointment at hospital.

Look at the following ways of transferring records. Which method is the most secure?

- by ordinary post
- by recorded delivery
- fax
- e–mail
- delivery by hand

Computer based records

Many hospitals and surgeries now keep records on computer.

The Data Protection Act (1984) covers all information that is held about people on computers. Every organisation that holds computer–based records must be registered, and there are guidelines for good practice that have to be followed.

1 The information must have been obtained legally and without deceit
2 The information should only be used for the purpose for which it was collected
3 The information should not be disclosed to anyone who has no right to see it
4 There should be a proper security system, with a password required for access

--- ● CASE STUDY ● CASE STUDY ● CASE STUDY ● CASE STUDY ● CASE STUDY ● CASE STUDY ● ---

Sarah works in a rehabilitation unit which has computerised records for all the patients. Sarah is updating the records on screen at the duty desk. A relative wants to speak to her about one of the patients. The details on the screen are clearly visible. What should Sarah do?

Giving and Receiving Information on the Telephone

We discussed this issue earlier in the chapter. With all phone calls dealing with personal information of patients and clients follow these rules:

- make sure the person asking for information has a right to know

- refer anything you are unsure about to your manager
- if taking a message related to personal details, make sure that the message is recorded correctly, and pass the message on quickly, ensuring that only the person who needs to know sees it. Messages may be folded or put in an envelope. Be careful about leaving confidential details on pieces of paper where anyone can see them

Future developments

With new technology, the NHS is developing a life long Electronic Medical Record of each patient, that can be accessed by GPs and hospitals. Some patients groups are concerned about confidentiality. Certain information will not be available to other professionals without the patient's consent. This includes:

- patients with HIV and AIDs
- patients who are on fertility treatment
- patients who have been treated for sexually transmitted diseases

PROMOTING AND SUPPORTING INDIVIDUAL'S RIGHTS TO DIGNITY, INDEPENDENCE, HEALTH AND SAFETY.

What do we mean by the term **RIGHTS?**
Think for a moment what you understand to be your rights.

➡ rights can be covered by laws e.g. the right to drive a car at 18, the right to vote, or get married
➡ rights can also been seen as natural or universal rights e.g. the right to work, the right to have children, the right to make choices about what you do in your daily life

In health and social care the rights of clients and patients are often stated in policies

---

THE RESIDENT'S BILL OF RIGHTS

■ to live a fullfilling life

■ to be treated with dignity as an individual

■ to have personal privacy for yourself, your belongings and your personal affairs

■ to do things at your own pace and when you want to do them

■ to perform any activity you feel capable of doing

■ to have your cultural, religious and sexual needs respected

■ to be free to make and keep contacts with the outside world

■ to be involved in decisions affecting your living arrangements

THE RESIDENT'S BILL OF RIGHTS (continued)

■ to associate with others and build up relationships

■ to have access to the facilities and services of the community

■ to take any risks implied by these rights without being unnecessarily restricted

■ to be consulted and involved in your personal care and to be given the daily care appropriate to your needs

■ not to be forced to do anything against your will

FIGURE 1.39 *The resident's Bill of Rights.*

Figure 1.39 is an example of a Bill of Rights for older people in residential care.

Most residential homes have a similar charter. You can find out about the rights of clients by looking at:

● codes of practice
● staff policies
● charters and other policies for service users
● standards of care
● individual care plans

CODES OF PRACTICE

There are many examples of Codes of Practice.

The UKCC (The United Kingdom Central Council for Nursing, Midwifery and Health Visiting) has a code of practice that covers all areas of patient care. Midwives have their own Code of Practice. This Code clearly states that *"in all circumstances the safety and welfare of the mother and her baby must be of primary importance".*

Local Authorities and Social Service departments also have clear Codes of Practice.

WHAT

We aim to help people stay in their own homes by giving them and their carers a wide range of support services. If it is no longer possible for you to receive care at home, we will arrange care in another place where you can keep your dignity and independence.

OUR

We have standards which you can expect us to meet when you write, phone or call in. We offer many services, and these are set out in our leaflet "Making Contact". There are also leaflets on standards for our other services and on how to make comments and complaints.

POLICIES FOR STAFF

Nowadays most organisations have a range of policies. These can include:

- health and safety
- equal opportunities
- confidentiality
- complaints policies and procedures

These policies give guidelines to staff, but also indicate how patients' and clients' rights should be protected

---

● *CASE STUDY* ● *CASE STUDY* ● *CASE STUDY* ● *CASE STUDY* ● *CASE STUDY* ● *CASE STUDY* ●

Norman is 75. He has Alzheimers Disease. He is a patient in a long stay unit for patients with dementia. Because of his condition, it is difficult to communicate with Norman. He spends the day time in the living area of the unit. There are 26 patients in the unit with dementia, and there are only 3 staff on duty. Norman is in a special chair, but he keeps rolling out of it and falling on the floor. The nurses are concerned he will fall and hurt himself, so they decide to tie him into the chair.

What is the problem here? How may this affect Norman's rights? Many organisations have a "restraint policy", which indicates when it is acceptable to secure a client so that they cannot harm themselves or others. It is important that staff follow the guidelines

CHARTERS FOR SERVICE USERS

Most organisations have developed Charters of Rights for clients. Figure 1.40 is an example of a Charter of Rights that has been developed by an organisation that assesses young people who have a physical disability.

The Patients Charter

The Patients Charter was developed by the NHS in 1995. It is currently being revised, so that certain standards will be set nationally and other standards will be set locally, in order to take account of regional variations.

The Charter defines two terms:

1 Rights

   These are what all patients will receive all the time.

2 Expectations

   These are standards of service that the NHS is aiming to achieve. Sometimes these standards cannot be met for exceptional reasons (e.g. a flu epidemic).

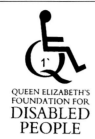

QUEEN ELIZABETH'S
FOUNDATION FOR
DISABLED
PEOPLE

CHARTER OF RIGHTS FOR RESIDENTS

As a resident of Dorincourt you should enjoy the following rights:

1. THE RIGHT to have your personal dignity respected irrespective of physical disability

2. THE RIGHT to be treated as an individual in your own right whatever your physical disability

3. THE RIGHT to personal independence, personal choice and personal responsibility for actions

4. THE RIGHT to undertake for yourself those daily living tasks which you are able to do

5. THE RIGHT to personal privacy for yourself, your belongings and your affairs

6. THE RIGHT to have your cultural, religious, sexual and emotional needs accepted and respected

7. THE RIGHT to the same access to facilities and services in the community as any other citizen

8. THE RIGHT to maintain and develop social contacts and interests

9. THE RIGHT to manage your own financial and private affairs

10. THE RIGHT to control your own medication and to make decisions about your medical treatment in conjunction with your own doctor

FIGURE 1.40 *Charter of rights of residents.*

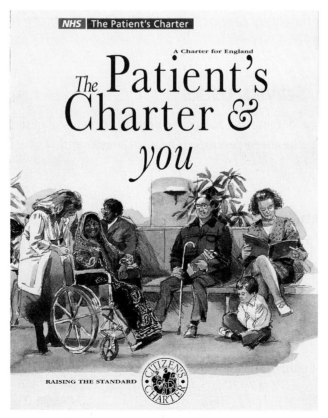

FIGURE 1.41 *Patient Charter leaflet.*

According to the Patients Charter as a patient you have the right to:

- receive health care on the basis of clinical need, not on ability to pay
- be registered with a GP and be able to change to another GP easily and quickly if you want to
- get emergency treatment at any time through your GP, the emergency ambulance service and hospital Accident and Emergency Department
- be referred to a consultant acceptable to you, when your GP thinks it is necessary and be referred for a second opinion if you and your GP agree this is desirable

When you register with your GP you have a right:

- to be offered a health check when you join a practice for the first time
- to ask for a health check up if you are between 16 and 74 and have not seen the GP for the last 3 years
- to be offered a health check in the GPs surgery, or at your own home if you prefer if you are 75 or over

Standards of Care

Local Authorities have contracts with voluntary and other independent organisations, and as part of the service agreement, the organisation has to provide care that reaches a certain standard.

Figure 1.42 shows an example of a Standards of Care statement.

PROVISION OF SERVICE/STANDARDS OF CARE

- to provide one to one bereavement counselling to clients from the age of 13 upwards

- to manage appointments, referral systems and maintain appropriate case notes

- to maintain a list of other statutory and voluntary agencies for referral if bereavement deemed inappropriate

- to ensure a high standard of counselling practice by effective use of training and supervision

- to continuously monitor the service provision, maintain accurate statistics and produce reports to inform our policies and procedures

- to assist and offer information and guidance to other statutory and voluntary agencies

---

FIGURE 1.42 *Provision of service/standards of care.*

Individual care plans

Care plans state what will be provided for a client, by whom, to whom, when, where and how. Care plans are drawn up with the carer, service user and the care worker. Care plans cover what the client has a right to expect. Care plans are reviewed at set times, as the care needed may change, and the care plan should be updated to reflect any changes.

Figure 1.43 shows an example of a care plan. Care plans are important written records and may be used in court, so they must be legible, clearly stated, signed and dated by the care worker.

CARE PLAN						Mrs Jones aged 64
DATE	NO	NEEDS/PROBLEMS	RATIONALE/AIMS	ACTION	SIGNATURE	DATE COMPLETED
5/10	1	Back pain (severe after fall)	Reduce pain	Bedrest, pillows in bed to support lower limbs, thermal pad applied		
	2	Overweight	Reduce weight	Consult dietician r.e. reducing diet		
	3	Depression	Reduce depression	Encourage Mrs Jones to read papers, listen to the tv/radio		

FIGURE 1.43 *Care Plan*

THE CLIENT HAS RIGHTS TO DIGNITY

When inspectors visit a home, they often use a check list similar to Figure 1.44.

Do residents have their own private room?	yes ☐	no ☐
Do residents have their own room key?	yes ☐	no ☐
Do residents have their own front door key?	yes ☐	no ☐
Can residents eat in private if they wish?	yes ☐	no ☐
Do care workers knock on doors before entering private rooms?	yes ☐	no ☐
And wait for an answer before entering?	yes ☐	no ☐
Can residents choose to be alone if they wish?	yes ☐	no ☐
Can a resident see a doctor in private?	yes ☐	no ☐
Do residents control their own money?	yes ☐	no ☐
Can residents go out when they like?	yes ☐	no ☐
Can residents attend any clubs outside the home?	yes ☐	no ☐
Can residents choose their own doctor?	yes ☐	no ☐

Do residents choose to be addressed by their first or surname?	yes ☐	no ☐
Can residents choose when to get up?	yes ☐	no ☐
Can residents choose when to go to bed?	yes ☐	no ☐
Are there staff/resident meetings to decide common interests/activities?	yes ☐	no ☐
Can residents arrange to eat at different times?	yes ☐	no ☐
Can residents make a snack for themselves or make a drink?	yes ☐	no ☐
Is there a choice of menu at meal times?	yes ☐	no ☐

FIGURE 1.44 *A quality checklist for residential homes.*

If the rights of residents to dignity are respected:

➡ staff will knock on the door before entering (and wait for an answer)
➡ staff will address clients by the name they choose
➡ the privacy of the client will be respected
➡ the client will not be asked to do anything that is embarrassing, and does not show respect to the individual

● CASE STUDY ● CASE STUDY ● CASE STUDY ● CASE STUDY ● CASE STUDY ● CASE STUDY ●

Mrs Holland is a resident who has newly arrived at The Cedars residential home. Before she retired she was headmistress at a well–known girls school. Mrs Holland is sometimes rather forgetful. She enjoys reading the Daily Telegraph each day. It is 8.a.m. and Mrs Holland is resting in her room. The door bursts open and Trudie, the care assistant appears.

Trudie. Ooh, love, I've had such a morning. I would have got to you sooner but we are short staffed today, and then Mr Brown on the landing had a "little accident". He didn't get to the loo in time and I had to clean him up. Oh well, we'd better get you ready for the bath. You do want a bath don't you?

Mrs H: Oh dear, I don't really feel like it today.

Trudie: Well I'm running the bath now, so we'd better undress you and get you in.

Mrs H: (struggling up and trying to undress) Oh dear.

Trudie: Come on then, I still have got the others to do. Shall I help you? (grabs Mrs Holland and starts undressing her) Come on love, I haven't got all day.

What do you think about Trudie and Mrs Holland?

● *CASE STUDY* ● *CASE STUDY* ● *CASE STUDY* ● *CASE STUDY* ● *CASE STUDY* ● *CASE STUDY* ●

Answer the following questions.

1   *Is Trudie respecting the dignity of Mrs Holland?*

2   *Is she giving her a choice whether on not she has a bath?*

3   *Do you think Mrs Holland likes to be called love by someone she doesn't know?*

4   *How would you feel if you were Mrs Holland?*

5   *Why might Trudie behave the way she does?*

6   *What might be done to support Mrs Holland?*

Discussion

One of the first things you should have noticed is how Trudie is discussing another client with Mrs Holland. This will make Mrs Holland wonder if Trudie discusses her with other residents. This is against principles of confidentiality.

Opening doors without knocking first shows a lack of respect for a person. Trudie speaks to Mrs Holland as if she is a child, and does not ask her how she wants to be addressed. Trudie could have offered a choice of a wash instead of a bath which can be a struggle for an older person. Perhaps Trudie does not realise what she is doing wrong; perhaps all the care workers behave in the same way in the home so that staff training is needed. Shortage of staff may mean that not enough staff are employed in the home and this can be stressful for everyone.

INDEPENDENCE

Clients and patients should be supported so that they can be as independent as possible. Independence is linked to:

● self respect

● responsibility

● being able to choose

● being an individual

When we are babies and young children, we are dependent on other people but when we grow up we become independent individuals, with our own ideas interests, friends and personal skills. If we become:

- patients in hospital
- physically disabled
- mentally ill
- older

we are still the same individual.

People who are born with either learning difficulties or physical disabilities are also individuals who should be encouraged to be as independent as possible. The word "care" should mean supporting someone to develop their full potential but often it seems to mean controlling someone.

Look at the 2 case studies and decide what type of support would help Imran and Bridget achieve independence.

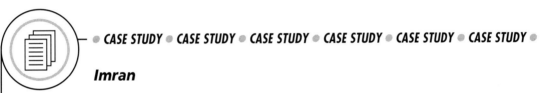

CASE STUDY ● CASE STUDY ● CASE STUDY ● CASE STUDY ● CASE STUDY ● CASE STUDY ●

Imran

Imran (aged 6) was knocked down by a car when he was out with his older sister. He suffered concussion and a broken leg, but is making a good recovery at home. His mother is very anxious about letting him go back to school in case someone knocks into him. She is also very worried about letting him go to stay with friends in case he has another accident.

Bridget

Bridget is 86. She has just come home from hospital, after falling and breaking her hip. She lives on her own. Her married daughter is determined that her mother will stay at home and not go out in case she falls over again. She wants her mother to have a panic button, meals on wheels, a shopping service and a home help. She is also making arrangements for a stair lift to be installed. Her mother is ignoring all these arrangements and insists she will go down to the town on the mini bus service.

As you can see from these examples, you will often find that relatives are so concerned about possible problems that they are restricting the independence of the person they are trying to protect. As a nurse or social worker, how would you try to encourage Imran and Bridget to develop their independence?

Promoting independence can involve risk. In some residential homes for all age groups, residents are encouraged to go out shopping, to the pub, to the local church etc. Depending upon the condition of the client, each activity could have a risk attached, and it is important that the care worker discusses risks with the relatives and client, and a decision is made whether the level of risk is acceptable.

We all take risks in our everyday life. Good care work is about supporting clients and patients to retain their independence and make choices about their lives.

Health and Safety

Health and safety is an important aspect in the hospital, residential home, day centre, or in the clients own home.

Figure 1.45 is a check list used in residential homes to assess health and safety. You could use this yourself at your work experience placement.

		COMMENTS	ACTION REQUIRED
Safe movement			
Are doorways, hall, stairs, landings and bedside areas well lit and free from clutter?	YES/NO		
Do doors and windows in all rooms (especially the bathroom) open and shut easily?	YES/NO		
Are any floors, stairs, steps, outside paths and all floor coverings damaged, uneven or slippery?	YES/NO		
Are all areas free from trailing flexes?	YES/NO		
Are firmly fitted handrails in use on both sides of the stairs, by the toilet and bath?	YES/NO		
Reaching			
Are shelves and cupboards in daily use in easy reach?	YES/NO		
Are heavy items stored on high shelves or on top of wardrobes?	YES/NO		
Can door butts, window catches, light switches, gas supply and post and milk deliveries be reached without difficulty reaching and stooping?	YES/NO		
Heating			
Are all fires and heaters adequately guarded and well clear of furniture, curtains and bedclothes?	YES/NO		
Are gas taps loose or are makeshift devices being used instead of proper gas connections?	YES/NO		
Are paraffin and bottled gas stored in a safe place in their proper containers?	YES/NO		
Are all rooms well ventilated?	YES/NO		
Are living rooms in daily use and bedrooms kept comfortably warm?	YES/NO		
Lighting			
Is there enough lighting for all concerned to safely negotiate stairs and passages?	YES/NO		

	COMMENTS	ACTION REQUIRED
Cooking Are all -pans and utensils in good condition? YES/NO		
Are there adequate uncluttered work surfaces besides the cooker and sink to avoid carrying hot pans around the kitchen? YES/NO		
Are tea towels dried over the cooker? YES/NO		
Electricity Are all electrical appliances flexes and plugs in good condition? YES/NO		
Are any adapters running two or more appliances from one socket? YES/NO		
Are there any electrical appliances in the bathroom apart from those specially adapted for bathroom use? YES/NO		
Are electric blankets in good condition i.e. dry, flat and regularly serviced? YES/NO		
Living and bedroom arrangements Are beds and chairs the right height for getting into and out of without strain? YES/NO		
Does the arrangement of furniture allow freedom of movement and does not create a fire risk? YES/NO		
Are mirrors hung over the fireplace? YES/NO		
Are hot water bottles dangerously worn? YES/NO		
Is there any other obvious hazzard, if so please specify? YES/NO		

Once the initial assessment has been carried out, it is the duty of all staff working within this environment to be alert and inform immediately their Manager of any changes to the above or any further hazzards.

FIGURE 1.45 *Health and safety checklist.*

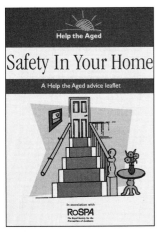

FIGURE 1.46 *Safety In Your Home leaflet.*

As a care worker you have a responsibility for the health and safety of yourself and of your patients and clients. In the hospital and clinic, there are special containers for the disposal of "sharps" that is, syringes and needles. Wet floors can be hazardous. Electrical appliances that are faulty should be reported.

Help the Aged has produced leaflets (see Figure 1.46) about safety in the home, especially for older people and children. Figure 1.47 shows the numbers of deaths from falls among people over 75.

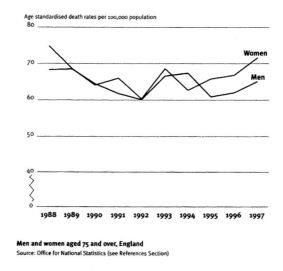

Men and women aged 75 and over, England
Source: Office for National Statistics (see References Section)

FIGURE 1.47 *Deaths from accidental falls in older people are not reducing*

What preventative measures can be taken?

Older people should be encouraged to keep active so that their mobility and balance is retained. Well lit areas in the home, well–fitting carpets and non–slip surfaces will guard against accidents. Bath mats and bath rails will protect against falls in the bathroom. Kitchen utensils should be kept in accessible cupboards so that the person does not have to climb on a chair to reach.

ACKNOWLEDGING INDIVIDUALS' PERSONAL BELIEFS AND IDENTITY

People' s values, beliefs and religion are part of their identity. Religious beliefs should be respected. The care worker can support the individual by:

● observing any dietary or other requirements

● respecting the wishes of the patient – for example by contacting the priest or minister if the patient requests it

In some cases, the treatment of the patient may include therapy that is not allowed by the persons' religion.

● *CASE STUDY* ● *CASE STUDY* ● *CASE STUDY* ● *CASE STUDY* ● *CASE STUDY* ● *CASE STUDY* ●

Sophia has just had her first baby. It was a difficult birth, and she lost a great deal of blood. The consultant wanted to give her a blood transfusion, but Sophia is a Jehovah's Witness and this religion bans the use of blood transfusions. The consultant could apply to the High Court to overrule Sophia's wishes. The risks to Sophia are explained to her and her husband and they remain adamant that they do not want a transfusion.

● *CASE STUDY* ● *CASE STUDY* ● *CASE STUDY* ● *CASE STUDY* ● *CASE STUDY* ● *CASE STUDY* ●

Heather is four months pregnant with her first baby. When she has a scan, the doctor realises the baby has serious deformities. A second scan four weeks later confirms the original diagnosis. Heather is offered a termination. She is a committed Roman Catholic and will not consider a termination. The doctor arranges for her to see a neonatal specialist, who discusses the level of disability with her. Heather continues with her pregnancy.

In both these situations, the role of the health and care worker is to give Heather and Sophia information about possible outcomes, so that they are making an informed decision, and to support them after they have made that decision. The care worker should not pass judgments or make critical comments on the decisions made by clients and patients.

SUPPORTING INDIVIDUALS THROUGH ALTERNATIVE APPROACHES TO COMMUNICATION

Clients or care workers:

● can speak different languages
● can have hearing loss or limited vision

Some client groups:

● may find it difficult to speak
● may have limited understanding

We can see that there can be difficulties communicating with different groups, but if we are going to deliver care according to the principles of the Value Base we need to be aware of how we can overcome these barriers.

Different languages

> ● **CASE STUDY** ● **CASE STUDY** ● **CASE STUDY** ● **CASE STUDY** ● **CASE STUDY** ● **CASE STUDY** ●
>
> *Midwives in West London discovered that very few Bangladeshi women were attending antenatal clinics, and this meant that sometimes problems with the pregnancy were not identified. A link worker scheme was set up. Bangladeshi women who had a good understanding of English were recruited, and trained. In specialist areas such as midwifery, it is important that the link worker is able to act as interpreter between the doctor or midwife and the patient, but the link worker also needs to have insight into the difficulties that may be caused by the difference in culture. Asian women tend to look away from a professional person as an act of respect, but the doctor may interpret this non–verbal communication as hostility or lack of interest. The link worker can act as a bridge between the two cultures.*

Mistakes that are made

● the health professional talks loudly to the patient, thinking this might help

● the health professional may try sign language which may add to the confusion

Communication barriers due to language problems means that

● the care worker becomes irritated and frustrated.

● the patient does not understand what is going on and cannot contribute to the discussion of care or future planning

Possible solutions

● use of interpreters in face to face situations, these can either be staff working in home or hospital, or relatives

● use of leaflets and other written information in the patients own language

The Patients Charter is available in many languages, and many hospitals are providing information in languages other than English.

It is difficult to cover all languages. In the London area alone, it is estimated that there are over 300 different languages spoken.

● use of Language line. This is a specialist telephone service that interprets phone calls. It is used by NHS Direct. Figure 1.48 shows an example of a leaflet giving advice in other languages

This leaflet is one of a series explaining what you can expect
from Sutton Council. If you would like a copy in your own
language, or more information, please contact xxx.

આ પત્રિકા, તમે સટન કાઉન્સીલ પાસે શું આશા રાખી શકો તને સમજાવવાની
શ્રેણીની પત્રિકાઓમાંની એક છે. જો તમને આની નકલ તમારી પોતાની ભાષામાં
જોઈએ અથવા વધુ માહિતી જોઈએ તો, મહેરબાની કરીને xxx
પર સંપર્ક કરો.

GUJARATI

یہ لیف لٹ اُن کئی اشاعتوں میں سے ایک ہے جو یہ وضاحت کرتا ہے کہ سٹن کنسل سے آپ کیا توقع رکھ سکتے ہیں۔ اگر
آپ اس کی ایک نقل اپنی زبان میں حاصل کرنا چاہتے ہیں یا اس بارے میں آپ کو مزید معلومات درکار ہیں تو براہ کرم
020 8770 5130 پر رابطہ کیجے۔

URDU

تعتبر هذه النشرة الإعلامية واحدة من عدة نشرات لتشرح لك عما تستطيع أن
تتوقع من بلدية «ساتون». إذا كنت ترغب في الحصول على نسخة مترجمة في
لغتك الاصلية أو لمجرد الحصول على المزيد من المعلومات، نرجو منك الاتصال
على رقم الهاتف التالي: 020 8770 5130

ARABIC

Kjo fletushkë është vetëm njëra nga seriali që ju spjegon se qfarë
shërbime mund të pritni nga kansilli i Sutonit. Poqëse dëshironi
një kopje në gjuhën e juaj amtare ose më shumë informata, ju
lusim që të na kontaktoni në numrin 020 8770 5130

ALBANIAN

我們有一系列小冊向你解釋你可對撒頓議會政府
有何期望，這只是其中的一份．假如你想索取中文的小
冊或更多資料，請打電話 020 8770 5130

CHINESE

**If you want a copy of this leaflet in
large print, Braille or on tape,
Please contact xxx.**

April 2000

FIGURE 1.48 *Example of leaflet in other language.*

Hearing loss

Approximately 3 in every 1,000 children are born with a hearing loss. The majority of deaf
children are born to hearing parents. The chance of having a hearing loss increases with age. It
is estimated that one third of people aged 60 – 70 and three quarters of all people have a
hearing loss.

UK	16–60 YEARS	OVER 60 YEARS	TOTAL
Mild/moderate deafness	2,213,000	5,754,000	7,967,000
Severe/profound deafness	102,000	571,000	673,000
All degrees of deafness	2,315,000	6,326,000	8,640,000

TABLE 1.5 *Estimated numbers of deaf and hard of hearing adults in the UK in 1996.*

Table 1.5 shows the numbers of people in the UK with hearing loss.

● At least 50,000 people are estimated to use BSL (British Sign language)
● At least 154,000 people lip read
● 21,000 people are both deaf and blind

- in some hospitals and residential homes there could be an interpreter who can sign (using BSL) so that communication between the care worker/professional is maintained
- many local adult education centres run classes for people to learn BSL
- RNID (Royal National Institute for the Deaf) gives useful information on learning how to sign

Figure 1.49 shows the basic alphabet for signing

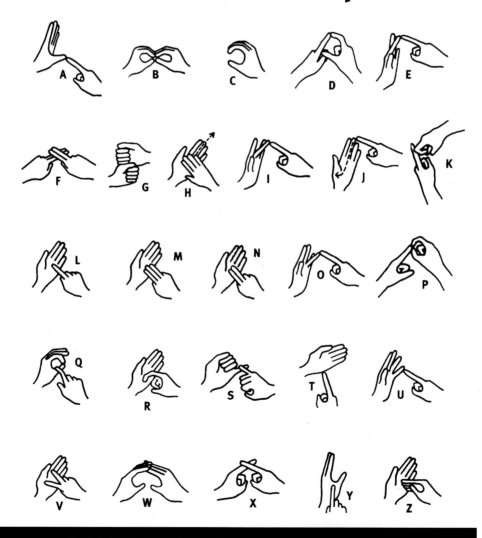

FIGURE 1.49 *The signing alphabet.*

LIP READING

Lip-reading is very tiring for the person lip reading.

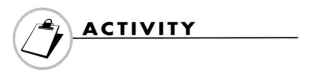

ACTIVITY

Next time you are looking at a news programme on the television, turn the sound down and see how much you can understand. You will notice that your understanding is helped if there are prompts, such as pictures, which gives you an idea about the subject.

Try the same activity with a friend, who is mouthing words rather than saying them and see how well you do.

Key points when talking to someone who is lip reading

- stand in front of the deaf person, 3 to 6 feet away and at the same level as them
- face the light rather than have the light behind you, as the person needs to be able to see your face clearly
- turn off television and keep background noise to the minimum possible
- check that the deaf person is looking at you before you speak
- do not shout, as this will distort your voice and lip patterns
- keep your head still, don't turn away
- don' t cover up your mouth with your hands
- do not eat while you are speaking
- gestures may help understanding, e.g. pointing to yourself or to what you are talking about
- do not switch from talking about one thing to another quickly
- write things down if you need to clarify them

Figure 1.50 is a useful way of remembering how to support people who lip read:

Research done by RNID in 1998 showed that visiting the doctor is very difficult for people who have a hearing problem.

The most common problems were:

1 Doctors not being able to communicate effectively with patients
2 Lack of interpreting facilities
3 Making an appointment

Can you think of possible solutions to these problems?

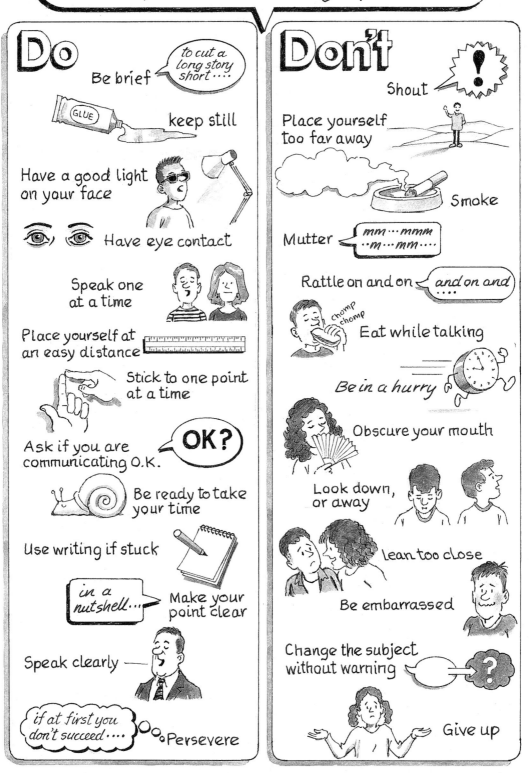

FIGURE 1.50 *Improving Communication Skills when working with people with hearing problems.*

Deaf Blind

In the UK it is estimated that 21,000 people are deaf blind. Communication is difficult with this group of people, as they cannot see non–verbal communication, as well as being unable to hear. Therefore touch is a very important source of communication.

Limited vision

Visual impairment can be due to a variety of causes.

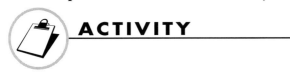 **ACTIVITY**

Working in pairs, take it in turns to be blindfolded. You could take the person who is blindfolded round the classroom or college. Afterwards discuss how you felt about the exercise, from the point of view of the carer and the person who was blind.

As a carer, you need to ask the person what is the most helpful way for them. If you cannot see, it is quite frightening if someone rushes up to you and grabs you by the arm. It may be more helpful, if the blind person takes the arm of the helper.

If you are working with a visually impaired person:

- introduce yourself, the person may not be aware of your presence
- sit or stand in the position that suits the blind person best
- reinforce your conversation with clear speech and touch the person if appropriate
- don't grab the person. Ask them if they need help to go somewhere and what help they need
- use tone of voice rather than facial expression to communicate mood and response
- do not rely on non-verbal communication
- make sure that information is transferred onto something that the person can hear such as tapes, if braille is inappropriate or not possible

Many blind people complain that much of the information about health and social care is in leaflets. Can you think of ways you could give information to blind people about the health services available to them?

If someone becomes visually impaired, for example, due to disease, the OT may visit the home and advise on ways of adapting cookers and other appliances so that the persons' independence is maintained.

Difficulty in Speaking

There are several groups of people that have difficulty speaking. This could be due to problems from birth, such as cerebral palsy, or difficulties in later life due to accidents or strokes. According to The Stroke Association, every five minutes someone in England and Wales has a stroke. Around 20,000 people each year have ongoing communication difficulties as a result of a stroke.

The Stroke Association runs programmes for people who have dysphasia (difficulty speaking) called dysphasia support. This involves a dysphasia support organiser working with specially-trained volunteers to help people with communication difficulties. Professional speech and language therapists also work with dysphasic patients. The Stroke Association also produces visual aids, (see Figure 1.51) that patients can use, so that they can communicate by pointing at the relevant picture.

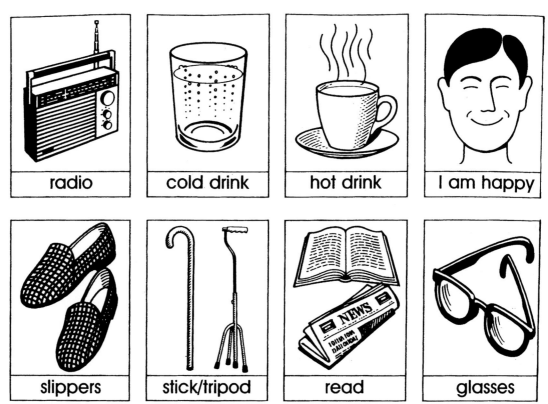

radio   cold drink   hot drink   I am happy

slippers   stick/tripod   read   glasses

FIGURE 1.51 *Communication board.*

When communicating with someone who has a speech difficulty, here are some do's and don'ts

1   do not finish the person's sentence for them
2   give them plenty of time
3   if you are not clear what they have said, ask them to repeat it
4   use picture cards, computers or other communication means
5   do not forget that the person can still hear, even if they cannot speak clearly

Limited understanding

There are at least two client groups you may work with who have limited understanding.

People with Learning Difficulties

People with learning difficulties can have different levels of understanding, so it is important that you identify the level either by speaking to a care worker, or by talking to the person.

- talk to the person at the right level, using words they understand and check they understand you
- repeat things so that you make sure they understand you
- respond to questions they ask you at the right level
- remain patient, and be prepared to take time over communication
- you can support verbal communication with drawings and diagrams

Makaton

Makaton is a language programme that has been developed for people with communication and learning difficulties. It was devised in 1972 by Margaret Walker, a Speech Therapist. It is used in the UK in pre–school settings, and in schools, day centres, hospitals and clinics, and in the homes of people with severe communication and learning difficulties. It has been adapted for use in 40 other countries. Many of the signs used in Makaton are from BSL. Makaton uses signs and facial expressions. Speech is always used with signs.

Figure 1.52 shows some of the basic signs. It is possible to learn Makaton at local education centres. Makaton has helped some groups to communicate effectively for the first time.

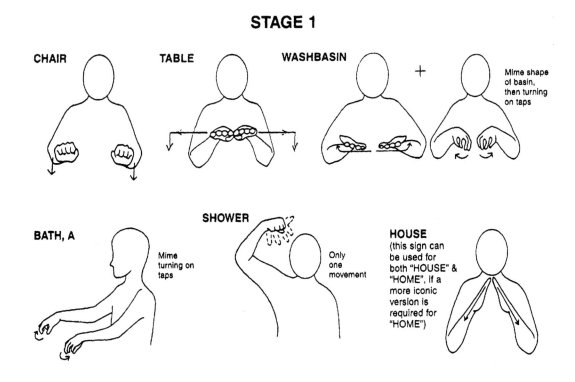

FIGURE 1.52 *Communicating using Makaton.*

Alzheimers Disease and Dementia

With dementia and Alzheimers Disease, communication can be affected because the client can suffer from short term memory loss, as well as confusion about time and place.

If you visit a residential home for people with dementia you may find that the staff make every effort to encourage the clients to be aware of time and place. There may be a board showing the day of the week and date. Photographs of recent events in the home may be displayed. Some activities may include "reminiscence therapy" when photos and past events are discussed. An example of this would be a scrapbook of local events during World War 2.

When talking to someone with dementia you need to:

Repeat information as often as necessary. This is because of the problems of short term memory loss, so you may be asked questions such as:

- What time is it?
- What is for lunch today?
- Where are we going?
- Who are you?

frequently, so it is important that you remain patient and repeat the information.

- keep conversation clear and simple
- use simple pictures or written information if this helps
- try to keep the patient in reality
- if the client says something strange, for instance a 77 year old says he is expecting to see his father that afternoon; do not assume he is confused but check the truth of the statement
- use distraction tactics if the client seems determined to do something dangerous to himself or others

Advocacy

This is when someone speaks on the behalf of someone else, who is unable to voice their views because of learning difficulties, mental health problems or other reasons. The advocate can be a professional, a volunteer or a relative. The advocacy movement developed in the 1980s when many of the large institutions closed and people were moved into the community. Because these people had become institutionalised and were unable to communicate their needs effectively, advocates worked on their behalf.

Peer advocacy

Advocates can be volunteers who have used the service themselves (in the case of mental health service users).

Skills needed by an advocate:

- honesty, sensitivity and discretion
- patience and perseverance
- commitment to assisting service users
- good communication skills
- ability to maintain confidentiality
- supportive to the client

People need advocacy in certain situations such as:

- admission to and discharge from hospital
- community care assessments
- care management arrangements (e.g. review of care plan)
- changes in treatment
- requests to see medical records
- complaints
- requests to change doctors
- important visits to GPs
- access to education and work

Apart from advocacy, where someone works on the behalf of the service user, there is also the development of **self advocacy**, where clients are supported and helped so that they can speak out for themselves.

In this section we have seen how communication methods can be adapted so that clients and patients can be supported towards a more independent life.

Word check

Empowerment

This term means the way in which a care worker encourages a client to take control of their own life, through effective communication of information to the client. The client is also supported so that they can take an active part in deciding how their needs can be met.

REFERENCES USED IN THIS CHAPTER

Bell, L. (1999) *Care Fully. A Handbook for Home Care Assistants.* Age Concern*

Carers in Employment (1995) The Princess Royal Trust

Crabtree H, and Warner L. (1999) *Too much to take on. A report on young carers and Bullying.* The Princess Royal Trust

Just the Job. Care and Community (1997) Hodder and Stoughton*

Just the Job Medicine and Health (1997) Hodder and Stoughton*

Just the Job. Nursing and Therapies (1997) Hodder and Stoughton*

Modernising Social Services White Paper (1998) HMSO

The New NHS Modern, Dependable (1997) DOH

Nolan, Y (1998) *Care.* NVQ level 2*

Richards J. (1999) *The Complete A – Z Health and Social Care Handbook.* Hodder and Stoughton*

Social Trends (1999) HMSO

Thomson, H et al. (1997) *Health and Social Care for Advanced GNVQ.* Second Edition Hodder and Stoughton

Thomson, H et al. (2000) *Health and Social Care.* Vocational A level. Third Edition

Thomson H. and Meggitt, C (1997) *Human Growth and Development for Health and Social Care*

Warner I, Wexler, S (1998) *8 Hours a Day and Taken for Granted.* The Princess Royal Trust

Wellards NHS Handbook 1999/2000 (1999) JMH Publishing

Worsley, J. (1998) *Taking Good Care. A handbook for care assistants.* Age Concern*

RESOURCES FOR STUDENTS

The references that could be useful are marked with an **asterisk** (*).

Most local authorities and local voluntary groups provide a range of materials that are relevant to the course. If you contact the head office of a national organisation, send a stamped addressed envelope and at least 60 pence in stamps to go towards the costs. You may find additional information on web sites, and these are listed under the Useful Addresses section.

The weekly publication Community Care has relevant articles. Local free newspapers usually cover health issues, and include examples of jobs in health and social care in the job advertisement section.

USEFUL ADDRESSES

If you write to organisations that are Charities, please enclose a stamped addressed envelope. Many of these charities and organisations have web sites and you may find it quicker to access the information you need through the internet.

Barnardo's
Tanners Lane
Barkingside
Essex 1GB 1QG

Child Poverty Action Group
1 – 5, Bath Street
London ECU9 PY

NSPCC (National Society for the Prevention of Cruelty to Children
National Centre
42, Curtain Road
London EC2A 3NH

Age Concern England
Astral House
1268, London Road
London SW16 4ER

Winged Fellowship Trust (Holidays for People with Disabilities)
Angel House
20 – 32, Pentonville Road
London N19 XD

Carers National Association
20/25 Glasshouse Yard
London CE1A 4JS

British Red Cross
9, Grosvenor Crescent
London SW1X 7EJ

The Stroke Association
CHSA House
123 – 127, Whitecross Street
London EC1Y 8JJ

Careers Advice

Degree Programmes in Nursing
UCAS
Fulton House
Jessop Avenue
Cheltenham Glos GL50 3SH

Health Service Careers
PO Box 204
London SE99 7UW
Tel: 0207 636 6287
Provides leaflets on different careers in the Health Service

NHS Careers
Tel: 0845 606 0655 (24 hours)
Website/e–mail: advice@nhscareers.nhs.uk
Advice on careers in nursing or midwifery

NHS Careers. PO Box 376
Bristol BS99 3EY
Contact for advice on minimum requirements for entry into nursing

NMAS
Rosehill
New Barn Lane
Cheltenham Glos GL52 3LZ
Tel: 01242 223707
For application package details for entry to nursing
Tel: 01242 544949 for general enquiries

Professional Association of Nursery Nurses
2, St James Court
Friar Gate, Derby DE1 1BT
Leaflets for nannies, setting up nurseries etc

Social Work Training
CCETSW
Information Service
Derbyshire House
St Chad's Street
London WC1H 8AD
web site: http://www.ccetsw.org.uk/england NF/start.htm

Glossary

Adoption – the legal transfer of an infant or child from the birth family to another family

Advocacy – in which someone speaks on the behalf of someone else, who is unable to voice their views because of learning difficulties, mental health problems, or other reasons. The advocate can be a professional, volunteer or a relative

Ageism – discrimination based on age, which means that a person is treated unfairly or differently from others because of their age

Alternative medicine (or therapy) – treatment of different conditions that focuses on the whole person (holistic) rather than just concentrating on the disease itself

Assessment – formal method of identifying the health and social needs of a service user in order to set up a care plan

Benefits Agency – the agency within the Department of Social Security which is responsible for the assessment and payment of social security benefits

Care plan – the plan of treatment and care decided upon jointly by the service user and the named nurse or key worker

Carer – person who takes on the responsibility for the care and support of a person who cannot fully support themselves

Case conference – formal meeting of professionals, service users, carers and family to plan future action

Charities – non-profit making organisations set up to support different groups

Child Health Surveillance Programme – system of development checks carried out in the first eight years of life

Chiropody – treatment of feet, also known as podiatry

Chiropractic – Alternative therapy involving manipulation of the spine

Clinician – any health professional who is directly involved in the treatment and care of patients (e.g. midwife, doctor)

Code of Conduct – professional code of behaviour and practice drawn up by a professional body to set standards (e.g. UKCC)

District Nurse – qualified nurse who works closely with the GPs and is employed by the Community Trust

Domiciliary services – health and social care services that take place in the service user's home

Foster care – care of child or children by the local authority in a family group. This can be provided by foster carers paid by the L.A, or by a fostering agency

Geriatrician – doctor who specialises in the diseases and disorders of older people

Health Authorities – regional and district – identify the medical needs of an area and manage the administration and development of health services

Health Improvement Programme – HimP – national, regional and local plans to improve the health of the population, focussing on particular needs relevant to the area

Health Visitor – a registered nurse with additional training, who works in the community to advise and support children under 8 and their families. The role has recently been expanded to include health promotion, including continence advice

Home Care Services – community team who provide social care for clients in their own homes

Homeopathy – alternative therapy using natural substances to help the body heal itself in a range of conditions e.g. eczema

Hospice – usually a small unit set up to care for the dying (terminal illness)

Independent Sector – agencies that provide health and social care independently from statutory providers. They can be private (profit making) or voluntary (non-profit making)

Informal care – care (usually unpaid) that is given by friends, family or neighbours.

Key worker – a named person who ensures that the care plan is followed and care is given to the client/patient. In health care, there would be a named nurse who is responsible for the care of certain patients

NHS Charter – Charter outlining the standards of care, including waiting times, patients can expect from the NHS

NHS Direct – a 24 hour phone service staffed by nurses

NHS Executive – Central management organisation in the NHS

NHS Trusts – hospitals or community services which are independent bodies and employ staff to deliver medical care

Occupational therapist – (OT) – therapist who treats patients in hospital and in the community and encourages independent living

Optician – professional trained to examine and test eyes, and prescribe lenses

Orthopaedic Specialist – surgeon specialising in the disease, injury and problems of bones and joints

Osteopathy – alternative treatment of muscles, bones and joints using massage, manipulation and other techniques

Paediatrician – qualified doctor who specialises in treating children

Pharmacist – qualified professional who dispenses prescriptions and gives advice to patients

Physiotherapist – professional who treats a range of conditions, including post operative rehabilitation, using exercise massage and other therapies

PCG (Primary Care Group) – set up in 1999 to deliver primary health care and to develop links with the secondary sector (hospital services) They will develop to become PCTs (Trusts) when they will commission and provide services in health care

PHCT – Primary Health Care Team – which includes GPs, nurses, pharmacists, opticians, and other health workers

Risk assessment – procedure that assesses the risks in the environment to the service user (e.g. unsafe home). It can also be applied to people with mental health problems when a doctor would decide whether the patient is a danger to himself or to others

Home service – when care workers and medical staff work together to support the patients in his/her own home

Secondary Services – medical care that is given in hospital rather than in the Primary Care setting

Self Advocacy – the service user is encouraged and assisted to speak on their own behalf about the services they need

Speech Therapist – professional trained to help adults and children overcome a range of problems related to speech and swallowing. Problems can include stammering, dysphagia (difficulty in swallowing) and aphasia (difficulty in speaking, for example after a stroke or head injury)

Tertiary care – medical care offered at a specialist hospital e.g. oncology (cancer) neurology (to do with the brain and spinal cord) or cardiac (heart)

ANSWERS TO ACTIVITIES

Types of Services

1 Informal

2 Statutory

3 Voluntary

4 Private

Bed Numbers Fig 1.8

Difference between 1982 and 1995

Total beds. 35,535 difference in total beds

1,250,000 more inpatients treated in 1995

1,748,500 more day cases in 1995

Carers

Figure 1.16

1 Spouse or partner

2 Friends/neighbours/other

Figure 1.17 Age of cared for

1 9 %

2 45 %

3 The figure is 13% lower.

Figure 1.19

Age of carer

1 17%

2 65 %

3 34 % or over 65 years of age

(figures do not add up to 100 %)

Children's Services Table 1.4

1 Health visitor
2 Speech and language therapist
3 Enuresis clinic
4 Community Dental service
5 Health Visitor
6 Audiology service
7 Community paediatrician
8 Child Psychiatrist
9 Educational Psychologist

Types of Questions Used in Health Care

1 Open Question
2 Closed Question
3 Multiple question
4 Biased question

Listening Skills Checklist

1 True
2 False
3 True
4 False
5 False
6 False
7 True
8 True

Should all patients be treated the same way? Figure 1.38

All patients should be treated as individuals. If you treat them all the same, you will not be showing awareness of the different needs of each person.

CHAPTER 2

Promoting
health and well–being

The knowledge and skills covered in this chapter will help when working with people in care situations.

After working through this chapter, you should:

➡ be able to define health and well–being

➡ know that aspects of health and well–being differ between different people and groups of people

➡ know about factors that affect health and well–being and the different effects they have on people

➡ understand physical measures that can be used to measure good health

Throughout the chapter there are activities to help you develop and test your understanding. Where appropriate, there are answers to questions at the end of the book. At the end of the chapter there is an opportunity for you to produce an assignment for grading; an explanation of key words and phrases, and a list of useful resources.

Definitions Of Health and Well–Being

'At least I've still got my health'. When someone says this, what do they mean by 'health'? It is likely that you understand their meaning, but it is difficult for you to define the word 'health'. Different people will have different ideas about health. There is a range of definitions of health and well–being used by ordinary people, professionals and different organisations.

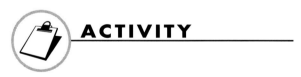

ACTIVITY

Before you read any further, think how *you* would define 'being healthy'. Ask a few of your friends what definition they would give.

Definitions from ordinary people

There are three states of health commonly identified.

1 **Negative definition**. Many people only think about health when they are thinking about illness or health problems. This means they may give a negative definition of health such as 'not being ill' or 'being free of pain'.

2 **The ability to function**. Some people think of health as the ability to cope with every day activities.

3 **Positive definition**. Some people think more positively of health as fitness and well being. They may associate health with moods and feelings, and a sense of balance.

 ACTIVITY

Read through the following statements, then match each person's definition of health with one of the three types of definition described above (i.e. negative definition. ability to function, positive definition.)

A A young mother who is just expecting her third child: 'To me, health is being able to cope with the children.'

B An elderly man: 'Health is when you haven't got any aches or pains and there's nothing wrong with you'.

C A twelve year old girl: 'I think that health is about feeling good. You feel strong and happy and relaxed.'

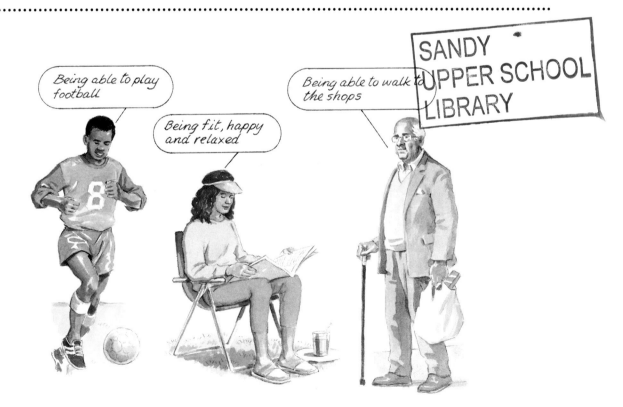

FIGURE 2.1 *Different standards of being healthy.*

People have **different standards** of what being healthy means to them (Fig. 2.1). This may depend on:

- **Age**: For example, a young person might only consider themselves healthy if they can take part in active sports, but an elderly person may consider themselves healthy if they can walk a short distance. From middle age onwards, people are more likely to think of mental well–being as well as physical well–being.

- **Sex**: More women than men include social relationships in their definition. For example, a woman is more likely to include meeting people, helping people, and having a good relationship with her family when talking about being healthy.

- **Lifestyle**: A smoker, for example, may not see a permanent cough as a sign of illness or an elderly person may think the loss of teeth is normal.

- **Class**: Studies have shown that middle–class people are more likely to think of health in positive terms, and working–class people are more likely to think of health in negative terms.

- **Where a person lives**: People living in an area where many children die within their first year and adults have a short life expectancy will have a different perception of health than people living in an area where death in childhood is rare and adults expect to life to a 'ripe old age'.

These examples show that ordinary people have a very **subjective** view of health.

 ACTIVITY

1 **A survey on the concept of health asked the following two questions:**
   (i) **Think of someone you know who is very healthy. Who are you thinking of? How old are they? What makes you call them healthy?**
   (ii) **At times people are healthier than at other times. What is it like when you are healthy?**
   Write down your answers to these questions and then ask a number of other people these questions and record their answers. Do their answers show that people of different ages have different ideas of what being healthy means?

2 **Read the statements in Table 2.1.**

• Free of pain	☐
• Coping with stress	☐
• Having shiny hair and a clear complexion	☐
• Rarely being ill	☐
• Living to an old age	☐
• Being slim	☐
• Being relaxed and happy	☐
• Able to play sports	☐

- Being able to think clearly ☐
- Having lots of energy ☐
- Being a non-smoker ☐
- Rarely going to the Doctor ☐
- Enjoying being with family and friends ☐
- Helping others ☐

TABLE 2.1 *Aspects of health.*

Adapted from 'Promoting health — a practical guide to health education' *What does being healthy mean? Tick if important.*
  (i)   **Tick all of those that are important to you.**
  (ii) **Choose the five statements which are the most important aspects of being healthy to you.**
  (iii) **Put these five in order, starting with the most important aspect.**
  (iv) **If you are working in a group compare your answers with others.**
  (v)   **Now think how an elderly person's answers may differ from yours.**
3 **Ask a person from each of the following categories to describe how they feel when they are healthy. (NB You will need to ask a parent or carer to describe a healthy infant.)**
  ● **Infant (0–3 years old)**
  ● **Young children (3–9 years old)**
  ● **Adolescents (10–18 years old)**
  ● **Adults (19–65 years old)**
  ● **Elderly people (65+ years)**

Make a poster to show the different attitudes to health with a photo of each person and a brief description of their view of being healthy.

DEFINITIONS FROM PROFESSIONALS AND ORGANISATIONS

The medical definition of health is often thought to be '**absence of disease**'. It does not describe health as a positive state. It views health as when you are not classified as sick or in need of medical help. It ignores the fact that health is about feeling well, energetic and at ease. It may also mean that people with disabilities or chronic conditions (see 'Key words and phrases') may be labelled as 'sick' or 'diseased' when they are otherwise healthy.

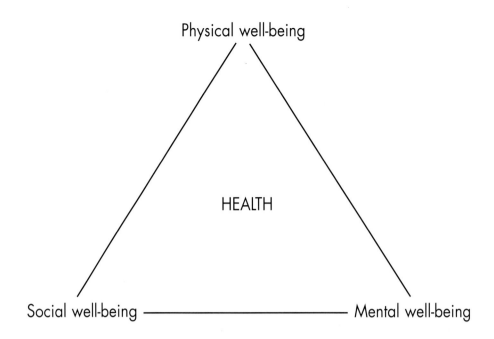

FIGURE 2.2 *WHO definition of health (1948).*

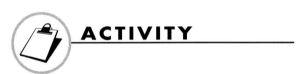 **ACTIVITY**

1 Look at the 'Key words and phrases' at the end of the chapter to check the meaning of illness; disease; and sickness.

   Think about occasions on which you have been unwell and decide whether thee episodes would have been classed as illness, disease, or sickness.

2 'Ordinary people' assess their health subjectively. Professionals assess health more objectively. What do you understand by 'objective' and 'subjective'?

A widely used definition of health came from the **World Health Organisation (WHO)** 9n 1946. This defines health as:

'a state of complete physical, mental and social well–being and not merely the absence of disease or infirmity'.

This has been widely quoted because it goes much further than just seeing health as freedom from disease. Instead health is viewed as all–round well–being (Fig. 2.3). However, it has been criticised for two main reasons.

● The first of these is that it is seen as too idealistic. How often do you really feel yourself to be in a state of 'complete well–being'?

● The second criticism is that it does not consider the ability to adapt to the changes that we all face throughout life.

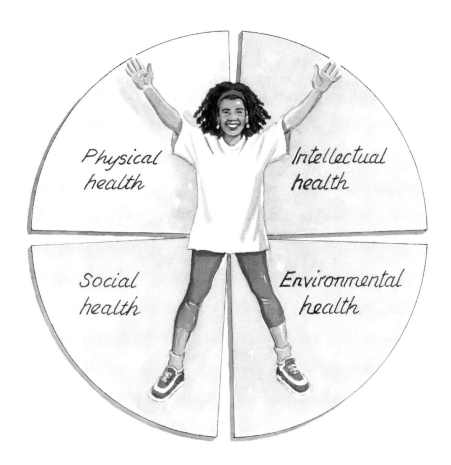

FIGURE 2.3 *The definition of health.*

In the light of these criticisms a more recent WHO definition of health is:

'the extent to which an individual or group is able, on the one hand, to realise aspirations and satisfy needs and, on the other hand to change or cope with the environment. Health is a positive concept emphasising social and personal resources as well as physical capabilities.'

This definition shows that:

- health is an important part of our everyday lives;
- it is a positive concept;
- health is a much wider concept than freedom from disease;
- health takes into account the whole person;
- health is related to our ability to cope and adapt to change;
- health might be understood in different ways by different individuals and groups.

PHYSICAL, INTELLECTUAL, EMOTIONAL AND SOCIAL HEALTH

The WHO definitions encourage the view of health as concerned with the whole person and not just their physical state. When thinking about a persons health you should think about physical, intellectual, emotional, and social aspects. You will be able to remember these if you think of the word 'PIES' (see Chapter 3).

➡ **Physical health.** This is concerned with the physical functioning of the body. Physical health is the easiest aspect of health to measure.

➡ **Intellectual health** (or **mental health**). This is concerned with the ability to think clearly and rationally. It is closely linked to emotional and social health (see below).

➡ **Emotional health.** This is concerned with the ability to recognise emotions such as fear, joy, grief, frustration and anger, and to express such emotions appropriately. Emotional health also includes the ability to cope with anxiety, stress, and depression.

➡ **Social health.** This is concerned with the ability to relate to others and to form relationships with other people.

You must remember that these different aspects of health are not separate but overlap and influence one another. For example, the pain and discomfort of an illness may make you unhappy. In this case, your physical health is influencing your emotional health.

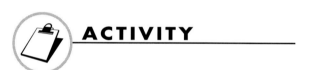 **ACTIVITY**

1 Look at the list of statements about being healthy in Table 2.1 above. For each statement, decide which aspect of health it is most concerned with — physical, intellectual, emotional, or social.

2 Read through the descriptions of the following people. Draw Table 2.2 and complete it by adding comments (for example, 'good', 'poor', 'not enough information available to comment') to show how you would assess each of the aspects of their health from the information you have.

ASPECT OF HEALTH	SHAZIYA	ANDREW	MARIE
● Physical			
● Intellectual			
● Emotional			
● Social			

TABLE 2.2 *Complete with comments on the different aspects of health (see case studies).*

● CASE STUDY ● CASE STUDY ● CASE STUDY ● CASE STUDY ● CASE STUDY ● CASE STUDY ●

Shaziya

Shaziya is a seventeen year old college student (Fig. 2.4). She is half–way through her Intermediate GNVQ Health and Social Care course. Recently she has been suffering from severe headaches which mean that she cannot think clearly enough to work on her assignments. This is putting her under a considerable amount of stress which she is finding difficult to cope with. She has a very supportive family and group of friends who are doing all they can to help her with these problems.

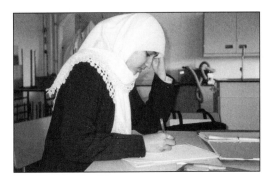

FIGURE 2.4 *Shaziya*

● CASE STUDY ● CASE STUDY ● CASE STUDY ● CASE STUDY ● CASE STUDY ● CASE STUDY ●

Andrew

Andrew (Fig. 2.5) runs a 150 acre farm single-handedly. Apart from the odd cold, he is rarely ill, and the nature of his work means that he is extremely physically fit. However, over the past few years, the crisis in the beef industry has caused his income to plummet and he is constantly worried because he has fallen behind with his feed bill payments. He does not mind the form–filling that other farmers often complain about, and keeps up to date with his 'paper work'. He rarely leaves the farm and has no close friends. His elderly father, who was his business partner for a number of years, recently went to live with his sister fifty miles away.

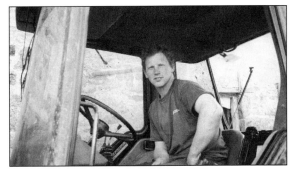

FIGURE 2.5 *Andrew*

● CASE STUDY ● CASE STUDY ● CASE STUDY ● CASE STUDY ● CASE STUDY ● CASE STUDY ●

Marie

Marie (Fig. 2.6 worked as a nurse in a a busy London hospital for a number of years until giving this up when she had her baby, Sam. Her partner works long hours and often travels around the country on business which means Marie is often alone with Sam. She misses her interesting work and rarely sees her friends. Because Sam often wakes in the night, Marie feels tired all the time. She spends a lot of time just sitting in front of the television, snacking on 'junk' food which has caused her to put on a lot of weight.

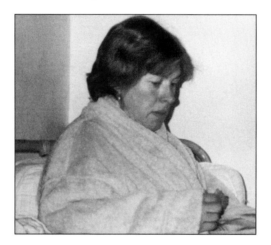

FIGURE 2.6 *Marie*

Factors Affecting Health and Well–Being

There are many factors which affect health and well–being. These may affect physical, emotional, social and intellectual health. You will be learning about the effects of the following factors:

● diet
● exercise and recreation
● environment
● social class
● employment
● housing
● income
● education

It is important to realise that the factors affect one another. For example, diet, housing and environment will be affected by income and social class. Income will be affected by employment. It is, therefore, difficult to identify the effect on health and well–being of one particular factor.

Diet

(see also section on diet under 'Risks to Health' on page 197 below)

A Balanced Diet

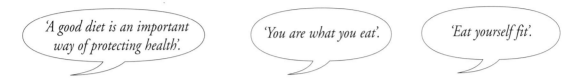

'A good diet is an important way of protecting health'.

'You are what you eat'.

'Eat yourself fit'.

These statements indicate the importance of diet to good health. A balanced diet has to contain the following:

- proteins
- carbohydrates
- fats
- fibre
- vitamins
- minerals
- water

Fig. 2.7 shows the relative amounts of the different food groups you should eat to have a balanced diet.

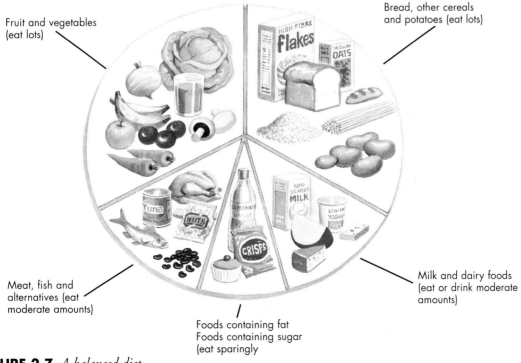

Fruit and vegetables (eat lots)

Bread, other cereals and potatoes (eat lots)

Meat, fish and alternatives (eat moderate amounts)

Foods containing fat Foods containing sugar (eat sparingly

Milk and dairy foods (eat or drink moderate amounts)

FIGURE 2.7 *A balanced diet.*

Proteins

Proteins are required for growth and repair. They are major components in the structure of enzymes (which control all the chemical reactions within the body), haemoglobin (which is the part of the red blood cells, which carries oxygen), and cell membranes. Meat, fish, cheese, eggs, nuts, grains and pulses are all good sources of protein.

Carbohydrates

Carbohydrates are the most important source of energy in the diet. Foods that are rich in carbohydrate are those which contain a lot of sugar, such as sweets and cakes, or those which contain a lot of starch, such as pasta, rice and bread. Because the 'starchy' foods release sugars more slowly and over a longer length of time into the blood, these foods are preferable to the 'sugary' foods.

Fats

Fats are a concentrated source of energy. They are necessary to provide us with fat-soluble vitamins, and they are an important component in cell membranes and some hormones. Plants tend to have liquid fats (oils) which are mainly *unsaturated*. Animal fats are solid at room temperature and are mainly *saturated*. (The terms 'saturated' and 'unsaturated' refer to the relative amount of hydrogen in the molecules. It is thought that an excess of saturated fat is particularly harmful to our health.)

Fibre

There is a type of carbohydrate, known as cellulose, which surrounds all plant cells. Cellulose cannot be broken down, so it remains undigested and is eliminated in the faeces. This fibre helps food to keep moving through the gut and prevents constipation. All fruit and vegetables are good sources of fibre.

VITAMIN	DAILY REQUIREMENT	MAJOR FOOD SOURCE	FUNCTION AND DEFICIENCY SYMPTOMS
A	100 µg	fish-liver oil, animal liver, dairy products (margarine contains added vitamin A); all green vegetables	needed for growth and functioning of surface tissues, especially those secreting mucus (deficiency leads to dry skin, mucous membrane degeneration)
			essential for vision (deficiency leads to night blindness, and eventually to complete blindness in children)
B vitamin (water-soluble)			
(B₁)	1.5 mg	widely distributed in plant and animal food (meat, wholemeal bread, vegetables)	essential for release of energy from carbohydrate (deficiency leads to beri-beri diseases, a form of nerve degeneration)
(B₂)	1.8 mg	widely distributed in foods, including milk	essential for release of energy from food

Vitamins

Vitamins are essential in small amounts in the diet for maintaining good health.

Minerals

We need 145 minerals (in organic salts) in our diet.

Water

Water is vital for health and is central to a balanced intake. A large proportion of food consists of water, and on top of this a person should aim to drink the equivalent of six to eight cups, mugs, or glasses of fluid a day.

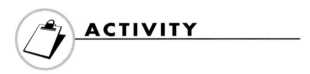 **ACTIVITY**

1 Find a book or website which shows the composition of a number of common foods. Which foods are good sources of:
   (i)   protein
   (ii) carbohydrates
   (ii) fats
   (iv) energy?
2 If possible, use a computer programme or internet website to analyse your diet and check that it is balanced. (see resources on page 223).

Recommended daily amounts of the different good groups

The amount of energy (in carbohydrates and fat), protein, vitamins and minerals required each day depends on factors such as our level of activity and age.

How much energy is needed?

Figure 2.8 shows the energy needs of different individuals. Look at the graph and list three factors which affect our energy requirements. (See end of Chapter for Answers.)

How much protein is needed?

The average UK diet provides more than enough protein: men generally consume 85 grams of protein a day, and women consume 62 grams. The recommended intake for an adult is 0.75 grams of protein per kilogram of body weight per day. (For example, a person weighing 70 kg would requires 0.75 × 70 grams of protein per day.) Some people, however, require additional supplies of protein, such as a growing children and babies; pregnant or lactating mothers; people who exercise heavily; people with viral infections, such as a measles, because protein is lost from their muscles, and is also needed for their immune defence; and patients who are recovering from illness or surgery.

ACTIVITY

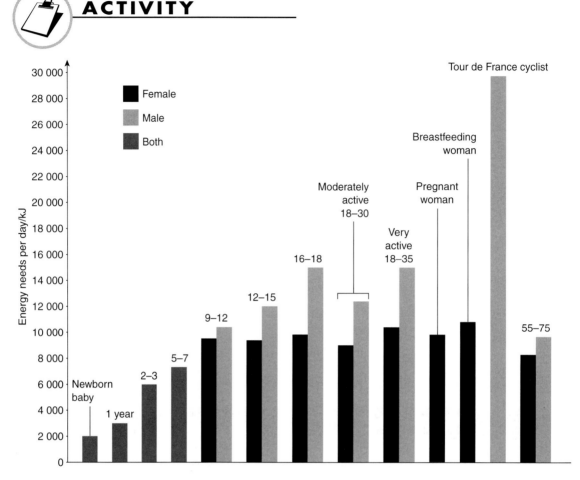

FIGURE 2.8 *The energy needs of different individuals.*

Healthy eating — Ten Top Tips

Because it is difficult for people to estimate whether they are having their recommended daily amounts of each type of nutrient in their diet, there are a number of useful guidelines worth remembering:

- No single food contains all the nutrients we need for health, so we need to eat a wide variety of foods each day.

- National and international targets have been set to encourage us to eat at least five 80 gram portions of fruit and vegetables every day.

- Eat lots of bread, other cereals or potatoes.

- Eat moderate amounts of lean meat, fish and alternatives.

- Eat moderate amounts of lower–fat milk and dairy foods (although children under 2 years old should not have reduced–fat milk.)

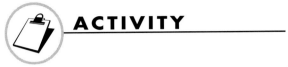

ACTIVITY

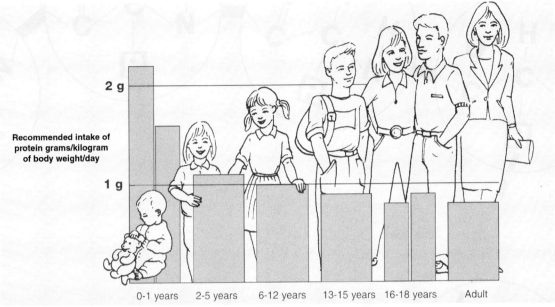

Recommended intake of
protein grams/kilogram
of body weight/day

2 g

1 g

0-1 years   2-5 years   6-12 years   13-15 years   16-18 years   Adult

FIGURE 2.9 *Protein requirements at various ages*   *Nestlé Worldview, Nestlé UK Ltd*

Use Fig. 2.9 to calculate how many grams of protein you should consume each day. (You will need to multiply the recommended amount from your age group by your body weight.)

- An average adult should drink about 6 – 8 cups of liquid a day. (For example, water, fruit juice, skimmed or semi–skimmed milk, or low sugar soft drinks.)
- Avoid eating too much fat and fatty food, particularly saturated fats.
- Eat foods containing sugar sparingly.
- Use a minimum amount of salt in cooking and try not to add additional salt.
- Healthy food needn't be boring. A balanced diet can contain chips and chocolate — it's just a matter of getting the balance right.

SPECIAL DIETS

The information above on recommended daily amounts of each type of nutrient shows that certain groups of people have particular dietary requirements.

Babies

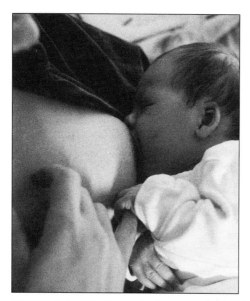

FIGURE 2.10 *Breast feeding provides all the nutrients a baby requires for the first few months.*

If possible, the best way to provide a baby with food is by **breast feeding**. Breast milk contains all the nutrients necessary for the first few months of a baby's life in the most easily digestible form. It will also protect the baby against some diseases as it contains antibodies, and may help to establish a close bond between the mother and baby. Breastfeeding is more economical and convenient than bottle feeding, as the milk is always at the correct temperature and there is no equipment to sterilise (Fig. 2.10.)

However, it is sometimes not possible for a baby to be breastfed, and the baby will be **bottle–fed with specially formulated baby milk**. It is important that this milk is made up according to the instructions n the tin or packet. It is recommended that cow's milk is not given to babies until they are at least one year old. **Solid food** can be introduced when the baby is between 4 and 6 months old, with breast feeding or bottle feeding continuing.

ACTIVITY

Product a leaflet or posted aimed at a new parent on one of the following topics:

● **Breastfeeding**
● **Bottle–feeding with formulated baby milk**
● **Introducing solid food into a baby's diet**

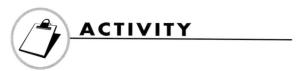

Children

It is particularly important that children have a well balanced diet because childhood is a period of active growth and development. There is also evidence that if a child develops healthy eating habits, these will last into adulthood. Children have a high protein requirement for growth (Fig. 2.9) and a high energy requirement relative to their small size. Their diet should be low in salt because their kidneys are unable to cope with high amounts. It can be difficult to feed 'fussy' children, but the following make healthy snacks:

- fresh or dried fruit
- raw vegetables like carrots
- bread or unsweetened biscuits
- unsweetened breakfast cereals (with milk, or dry)
- pop corn

 ## ACTIVITY

Young children are particularly susceptible to food allergies.

(i) Find out which foods most commonly cause allergies and what action can be taken. (See end of Chapter for Answers.)

(ii) If possible informally interview someone who suffers from a food allergy and find out how this affects their diet.

Pregnant and breastfeeding women

In the womb the developing baby obtains all its nutrients from the mother. It is, therefore, very important that she has a balanced diet. However, if the mother's diet is lacking in some way, this is more likely to harm the mother's health than the baby's health. For example, if the mother's diet lacks iron, the mother will become anaemic but the baby will not. If the mother's diet lacks calcium, the baby's bones will develop normally, but this will use up much of the calcium in the mother's bones, causing them to become softer, or even bent.

A woman should gain only 9–13 kg during the whole of her pregnancy. This means that while pregnant there is no need for her to eat more than usual. What is important is that she takes care to eat a balanced diet. It is necessary for pregnant women to have adequate fibre in her diet, because the hormones produced in pregnancy may lead to constipation.

Women need a higher level of extra nutrients when they are breastfeeding, than when they are pregnant. For example, they require more protein, vitamins and iron. The fat which accumulates in the woman's body during pregnancy can be broken down to produce some of the extra energy needed for milk production, but they will also need a more energy rich diet.

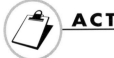 ## ACTIVITY

1   There is currently a debate about whether the government should make it compulsory for folic acid to be added to all manufactured bread and cakes. High levels are required in the first month after conception to prevent babies being born with neural tube defects, such as spina

bifida. It may also cut heart disease, and there are no apparent harmful side effects. If you have the opportunity divide into two groups (one for compulsory addition of folic acid, and one against), spend some time preparing your arguments, and then debate the issue.

2 If possible speak to a mother who has breastfed her baby. Find out if her normal diet changed when she was breastfeeding. For example, did she have a higher calorific intake?

The elderly

As people get older their energy requirement drops, partly because their metabolic rate decreases, and partly because they are likely to exercise less. However, it is important that the diet is not neglected in old age and that, even if the quantity eaten decreases, the quality and nutrient content of food remains high. Vitamin C deficiency is quite common in this age group due to a lack of fresh fruit and vegetables in the diet.

 ACTIVITY

List the reasons you can think of for why older people may neglect their diet. (See end of Chapter for Answers). Suggest ways in which the elderly could be encouraged to eat a healthy diet.

Exercise and Recreation

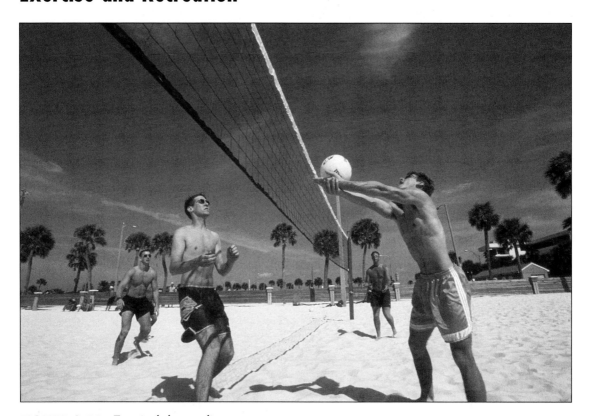

FIGURE 2.11 *Exercise helps to relieve stress*

Regular exercise and recreation can have a very position effect on health at any age. Some of the physical effects of exercise are listed below, but it should be remembered that any recreation undertaken in a group can also be good for a person's social health, and that exercising can lift feelings of mild depression, improve self–esteem, improve alertness and reduce stress (Fig. 2.11). The degree to which physical activity affects the body depends on:

● the type of exercise and how vigorous it is
● the duration of the exercise
● the number of times a week the exercise is repeated
● how fit the person is already

The latest research shows that 30 minutes of brisk physical activity five times a week are needed to improve health. This means any activity which makes you slightly out of breath. People who are not used to exercise should start with less and gradually build up to this.

PHYSICAL EFFECTS OF EXERCISE

● the heart becomes more efficient
● blood volume, red cells and haemoglobin increase
● arteries grow larger
● diaphragm grows stronger
● lungs become more expandable and increase in volume
● co–ordination improves
● the muscles and tendons can be stretched more easily, thus increasing flexibility of joints
● muscles increase in strength
● obesity is prevented
● the immune system produced more white blood cells to help fight infection
● the chances of developing conditions like arthritis, high blood pressure, diabetes, stroke, osteoporosis (brittle bone disease) or heart disease later in life are reduced
● the effects of ageing are reduced

Children and exercise

The amount of exercise children take has declined over recent decades. This has been caused partly by the increase in the amount of television watched, and partly because parents allow children to play outside less because of the increase in the amount of traffic. It should be remembered that taking part in games and sports helps children to develop friendships and self esteem, and so has a positive effect on their social, emotional, and intellectual health, as well as on their physical health. It is important that children have positive role models. For example, it has been found that more active parents tend to have more active children.

Teenagers and exercise

During adolescence physical activity declined by almost 50%, with females reducing their exercise levels even more than males. By the time they are 18, fewer than 12% of people take enough exercise to be considered fit.

Pregnant women and exercise

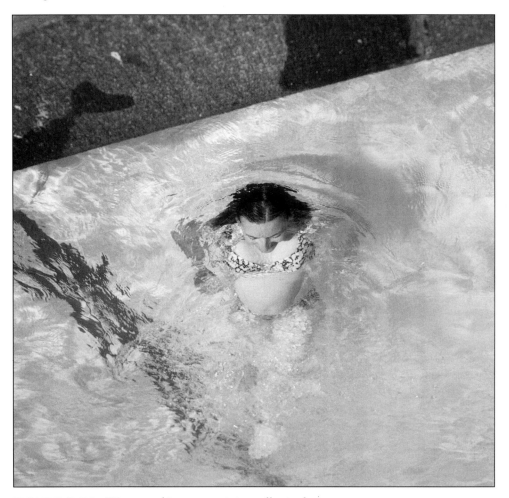

FIGURE 2.12 *Water aerobics – an activity well suited to pregnant women.*

Studies have shown that exercising during pregnancy is beneficial to the woman's health, and does no harm to the baby. It can reduce the mother's discomfort, tone the muscles in preparation for childbirth, improve her emotional health, and help with the control of weight gain (Fig. 2.12). However, the following precautions should be taken by pregnant women:

- Check with your Doctor before starting an exercise programme.

- Exercises at moderate intensity for 20 to 30 minutes at least three times a week.

- Don't exercise on your back after the first three months. This could reduce blood flow to your and your baby's heart.

- Avoid sudden–stop sports like tennis, or sports in which you may fall.

- Call your Doctor if you feel faint, sick, short of breath, or have abdominal pain, or vaginal bleeding.

Elderly people and exercise

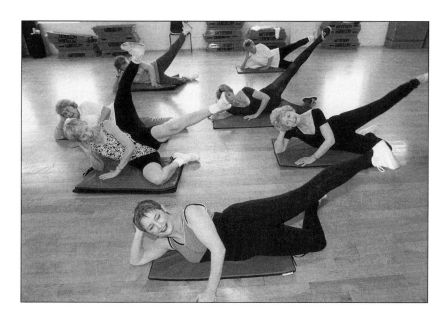

FIGURE 2.13 *You're never too old.*

Exercise is effective in slowing down the physical decline associated with ageing. For example, elderly people who exercise have significantly lower blood pressure, and better balance than those who do not exercise. They also sleep better. Swimming is considered a particularly good exercise because it works every muscle in the body without stressing joints. Some elderly people take part in very active sports, but it should be remembered that effective exercise can even be taken when sitting in a chair. Exercise done as a member of a group, can have a positive effect on physical, social, emotional, and intellectual health (Fig. 2.13.)

Individuals with special needs

People with disabilities can take part in a wide variety of sports (Figure 2.14).

Danger: too much exercise!

Many athletes train at a level which is harmful to their health. If too much exercise is undertaken, there is a higher risk of sports related injuries, and research has shown that there may be a higher rate of infection. Very intensive exercise can delay puberty. Some people are thought to become addicted to exercise, which means that lack of physical activity will have an adverse effect on their mental health.

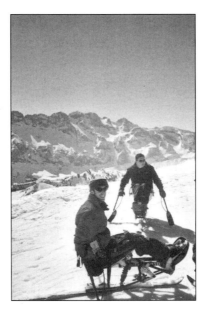

FIGURE 2.14 *People with disabilities can take part in a wide variety of sports.*

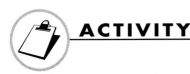

1 Look at the recommended amount of exercise above (5 × 30 min. each week). If you are not already doing this amount, plan activities that you would enjoy doing and how you could fit these into your week. (NB. Even short bursts of activity for 10 minutes, or so, add up to make a significant difference to your fitness).

2 Find out if there are any exercise classes in your area aimed specifically at the elderly.

If you go out on Work Experience to a local day or residential centre for the elderly find out what opportunities for exercise are offered.

Environment

The environment can be defined as our surroundings. As this is such a general term, it is often useful to consider a particular aspect of our environment. For example:

➡ **natural environment** (e.g. water, air)

Pollution of either air or water can have a marked effect on physical health, and noise pollution can affect all aspects of health.

➡ **public environment** (e.g. parks, museums, libraries, restaurants)

The public environment provides leisure opportunities. Leisure is essential for individuals to lead a healthy, balanced life. It encourages social contact outside the home, and many activities are concerned with fitness.

➡ **working environment**

(See section on 'Unsafe practices in the work place on page 208).

➡ **home environment**

(See section on 'Housing' on page 180, below).

Social Class

WHAT IS SOCIAL CLASS?

Social class is used to indicate the economic and social circumstances of an individual. There are different ways of defining which social class a person belongs to, but usually it is measured in terms of **occupation**. Table 2.3 gives the most recent classification of social class which will come into use in 2001.

- no account has been taken of relative earnings
- occupations have been sorted on the basis of factors such as job security and promotion opportunities
- a category has been added to include those who have never had employment and the long term unemployed.

HOW DOES CLASS AFFECT HEALTH?

As the statistics below show, the social class to which we belong may have long–term implications for our health and well–being. This is mainly because of the link between class and poverty. (See sections on Employment, Housing, and Income below).

- Men from the highest social classes have a life expectancy of five years more than men from the lowest social classes.
- In the lower social classes the death rates of men are higher than they were 20 years ago.
- Men from the lowest social class have death rates from coronary heart disease three times higher than men from the highest social class.
- A women from the lowest social class is twice as like to die before the age of 60 as a woman from the highest social class.
- A child born to parents from the lowest social class is twice as likely to die as a child from the highest social class.
- Children from the lowest social class are four times more likely to suffer accidental death than those from the highest social class.

What are the reasons for the health inequalities between the different social classes?

1 **Poverty** It is likely that people in lower social classes will have less regular employment and a lower income than those in higher social classes. This will mean they probably have a poorer diet and housing, both of which lead to poorer health (See sections on Employment, Housing, and Income, below).

2 **Poor access to the knowledge and resources that maintain health** Health education messages are less likely to reach people in the lower social classes. They are also likely to have lower NHS resource allocation.

3 **Poor working conditions** Manual workers have a higher level of diseases associated with hazards such as chemicals, dust and noise. They are also more likely to have accidents at work and to suffer higher stress brought on by carrying out boring, repetitive tasks.

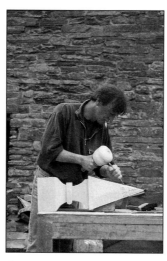

FIGURE 2.15 *There is a correlation between social class and smoking.*

4 **Smoking** The lower a person's social class, the more likely they are to smoke. For example, manual workers are more than twice as likely to smoke than those from the professional classes. Suggested reasons for this are:

- People from lower social classes are influenced more by advertising than by Health Education messages
- People from lower social classes are likely to suffer more stress which they attempt to counteract by smoking.

Incorrect assumptions can easily be made when discussing social class and health. For example, 'victim–blaming' is when health differences between people are dismissed as being 'their own fault'. For example:

➡ women from the lowest social classes are more likely to have low birth–weight babies who are less likely to survive.

➡ women from the lowest social classes are less likely to use the full range of ante natal services.

Looking at these two facts, a student commented '*If these mothers could be bothered to attend ante natal clinics and classes more, the babies' birth weights would increase, leading to an increased survival rate.*' However, this opinion is far too simplistic. It must be remembered that there are many reasons why these mothers may be less able to take advantage of ante natal services. For example, public transport may be poor; the woman may be in a poorly paid temporary job and her employers may ignore the legislation that requires them to give her time off for ante natal care; she may have a number of children for whom she cannot arrange care. It must also be remembered that there are a large number of other factors affecting the babies' birth weight. For example, poverty may mean the mothers have a poorer diet during pregnancy. They are more likely to have sub–standard housing and to have less opportunity for adequate rest and exercise.

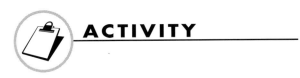 **ACTIVITY**

1 Do you consider that you belong to a particular social class? If so, which one? What are your reasons for your decision?

2 Read the information on 'victim blaming' above, then read the two facts below.

● People from the lowest social classes suffer more ill health than those from the highest social classes

● People from the lowest social classes eat more fatty foods and take less exercise than people from the highest social classes

Discuss

i) what prevents people from lower social classes from having a more healthy diet and taking more exercise; and

ii) what factors other than diet and exercise will cause their ill health? (See end of Chapter for Answers.)

3 Two suggestions are given above for the increase in smoking amongst people from lower social classes compared with those from higher social classes. Do you agree with these, and can you suggest others?

1. Higher managerial and professional occupations		2. Lower managerial and professional occupations	3. Intermediate occupations
1.1 Employers and managers in larger organisations: Company directors Corporate managers Police inspectors Bank managers Senior civil servants Military officers	1.2 Higher professionals Doctors Barristers and solicitors Clergy Librarians Social workers Teachers	Nurses and midwives Journalists Actors and musicians Prison officers Police Soldiers (NCO and below)	Clerks Secretaries Driving instructors Computer operators Telephone fitters
4. Small employers and own account workers	**5. Lower supervisory, craft related occupations**	**6. Semi-routine occupations**	**7. Routine occupations**
Publicans Play group leaders Farmers Taxi drivers Window cleaners Painters and decorators	Printers Plumbers Butchers Bus inspectors TV engineers Train drivers	Shop assistants Traffic wardens Cooks Bus drivers Hairdressers Postal workers	Waiters Road sweepers Cleaners Couriers Building labourers Refuse collectors

TABLE 2.3 *Where you rate in the new social order.*

Employment

Ill–health can result from the stress and/or poverty caused by:

- unemployment
- job insecurity (the threat of being made unemployed)
- low wages

There is a lot of evidence to show that people in employment have better health and well–being than those who are unemployed. The following have all been found to be higher amongst the unemployed:

- death rates
- amount of long–term illness
- disability
- psychological illness
- risk of suicide
- stomach ulcers

(NB. Employment will obviously affect income, housing and diet so read the sections on these topics to find out how they influence health.)

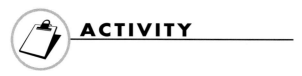 **ACTIVITY**

1 In January 1999 1.31 million were unemployed, the lowest figure for 18 years. Find out the current number of unemployed. How does the unemployment rate vary in different regions of Britain?

2 If you have experience of employment, write down what you gained from this, other than pay. If you have not been employed, informally interview people who are, and ask them how they feel they benefit from employment, other than financially.

   (See end of Chapter for Answers.)

Housing

It is difficult to know to what extent poor housing affects health. This is because people who live in unhealthy homes usually suffer from other forms of social disadvantage, such as poor diet, unemployment or poor education. A recent report by the Royal Institution of chartered surveyors concluded that thousands of people are killed every year by poor housing. Most of the 1.5 million homes which are officially classed as 'unfit for human habitation' are occupied. Poor housing is not only a problem in urban areas. In rural areas low wages and high unemployment mean that it can be difficult for young people to afford accommodation.

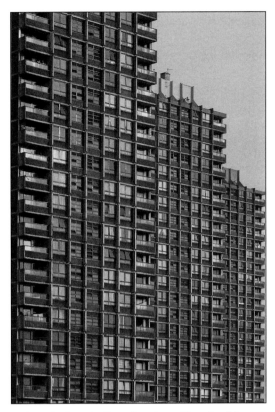

FIGURE 2.16 *Poor housing affects health.*

Characteristics of poor housing that have a direct effect on health:

- **Faulty design** may contribute to fires and falls in the home. The major location of house fires is in poor and inadequate housing. Children from the lowest social class are 16 times more likely to die in a house fire than children from the highest social class

- **Inadequate lighting** can be linked to falls.

- **Damp** is related to the growth of moulds and mites, and thus linked to respiratory diseases such as asthma. It is estimated that over 2.5 million homes in the UK suffer from severe dampness.

- **Inadequate heating** may lead to hypothermia, particularly in the elderly. The poorest usually live in badly insulated homes which are the most expensive to heat.

- **Overcrowding** can lead to the spread of infectious diseases, such as TB, and an increase in the incidence of stress and mental illness.

- **Poor sanitation**, for example, the shared washing facilities in bedsits and bed–and–breakfast hostels, can lead to the spread of disease.

- **Inadequate food storage and cooking facilities** increase the incidence of food poisoning and make a poor diet more likely.

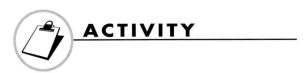

ACTIVITY

1 Read the following account of a young mother's living conditions. Write a list of the health problems she and her young child have, and for each suggest how these may have been caused by aspects of their housing. (See end of Chapter for Answers.)

Sally lives with her child, Sam, in bed–and–breakfast accommodation. They have one room and share a kitchen, toilet and bathroom with two other families. Their room is on the second floor which makes life difficult as Sam is still in a push chair. In their room there is a problem with damp in the winter, and this is made worse because Sally has to dry their clothes on the radiator. There are no nearby food shops, so she often relies on fish and chips from the mobile food van that visits. When she leaves food in the shared fridge it often disappears, so she keeps most of her food in the bottom of her wardrobe. Sally gets fed up with all the rules:- children aren't allowed to play in the corridor; there is no hot water after 10 pm; the kitchen is locked at 9 pm; no visitors are allowed. Since they have lived there, Sam has frequently suffered from asthma, Sally occasionally has a bad back, and they both sometimes have diarrhoea. Recently Sally has been feeling depressed.

2 There is a high incidence of mental illness amongst homeless people. Discuss whether you think mental illness leads to homelessness, or whether homelessness leads to mental illness.

Income

As mentioned in the sections above, there is a strong link between poverty and health. This is because the level of a person's income will affect their diet, environment and housing.

The Government Poverty audit includes people in households where the entire family income is less than half the national average household income. This is currently 12 million people, or 24% of the population. (This has risen from 5 million people in 1979.)

- A single adult is considered to be living in poverty is s/he has an income of less than £73.50 per week (after housing costs)
- A couple with no children are considered to be living in poverty if they have an income of less than £133.50 per week (after housing costs)
- Two adults with three children are considered to be living in poverty if they have an income of less than £223 per week (after housing costs)

Certain groups face especially high risks of poverty. In the UK a third of children, half of the lone–parent families, about 40% of pensioners, and about 70% of families where the breadwinner is unemployed live in poverty.

There is evidence to show that it is not just poverty that has a harmful effect on health. 'Relative poverty' means being poor in a rich society, and it is thought that this has the worst effect on health. Societies with small differences between incomes have lower death rates than societies with large differences between incomes. It is, therefore, worrying that in the UK the gap between the people with the lowest incomes (mainly pensioners, children and women) and the people with the highest incomes is growing.

- The poorest 10% of the population have incomes no higher than they did virtually two decades ago.
- Over the same period the income of the richest 10% grew by one half.
- The gap between those with middle incomes and both higher and lower incomes has also grown.

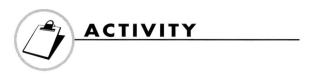

ACTIVITY

1 **In 1999 a minimum wage was introduced by the Government. Find out the current minimum wage, and then in a group discuss:**

   Has the minimum wage been set at a reasonable level?

   What are the advantages and disadvantages of setting a minimum wage?

   (See end of Chapter for Answers.)

2 **Read the following quote and then discuss whether you agree with it, and if so, why:**

   "The way to reduce ill health in impoverished areas is to reduce poverty. The most important steps any government can take are to increase the incomes of those on income support, to increase child benefit, to guarantee high quality pre–school education, and to reduce real rents in housing. Social expenditure is likely to have more effect in the long term than health expenditure."

Education

Education has been said to be 'the one way out of the dismal mixture of poverty, unemployment and crime.' People with very low literacy are much more likely to be classified as depressed as those with good basic skills. It is, therefore, unfortunate that poor children are more likely to have trouble with their education than children from higher income families (see Figure 2.17.) Good education can improve health on two fronts.

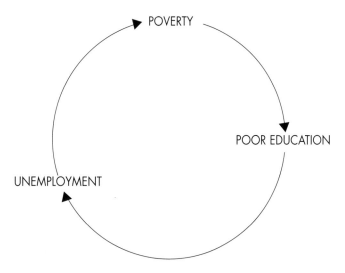

FIGURE 2.17 *The loop of poverty and poor education.*

It can inform pupils and students about health related topics such as diet, and teenage pregnancy, and it can improve a person's chances of employment, and therefore, make them less likely to suffer from poverty.

 ACTIVITY

1   **In 1997 the Government Minister for Public Health said schools could do more to help health and well–being. It was suggested that schools should develop a 'healthy school' philosophy and, for example, put more emphasis on supplying healthy school meals, and reducing teenage pregnancies.**

    In what ways do you think your school or college helps its students' health and well–being?

    In what ways do you think your school or college could do more to help its students' health and well–being?

2   **The Minister for Health also said " Teenage pregnancy is all too likely to be a cause as well as a symptom of poor education, unemployment and social exclusion. If a healthy school can keep a child from following her mother by getting pregnant at 17, she has a better chance of getting qualifications, getting a job, and breaking out of the loop."**

How do you think teenage pregnancy can cause poor education? (See end of Chapter for Answers.)

Do you agree that teenage pregnancy is likely to be a symptom of poor education (i.e. that a girl with a poor education is more likely to get pregnant as a teenager than a girl who has received a better education)?

Risks to Health

As you will have seen from the above information, a person's health can be affected by a number of factors. Some of these factors people may have little control over, but others are a matter of personal choice. People can put themselves at risk because of what they choose to do, or not to do. The health risks explained here include those that can result from:

- substance abuse, including legal and illegal drugs
- diet
- stress
- personal hygiene
- lack of physical exercise
- sexual behaviour
- unsafe practices in the workplace

USE OF ILLEGAL DRUGS

Illegal drugs are those whose non–medicinal use is banned by the Misuse of Drugs Act. Table 2.4 gives information on the most commonly used of these. The Misuse of Drugs Act places banned drugs in different classes, A, B and C. Offences involving Class A drugs carry the highest penalties; offences involving class C drugs the lowest.

Facts about drugs

	other names include	what it looks like & how it is taken	the effects	the health risks	legal status
ALKYL NITRITES	poppers amyl nitrite, butyl nitrite, isobutyl nitrite product names include: Ram, Thrust, Rock Hard, Kix, TNT, Liquid Gold	• clear or straw-coloured liquid in a small bottle • vapour which is breathed in through the mouth or nose from a small bottle or tube	• brief but intense 'head-rush' • flushed face and neck • effects fade after 2 to 5 minutes	• headache, feeling faint and sick • regular use can cause skin problems around the mouth and nose • dangerous for people with anaemia, glaucoma, and breathing or heart problems • if spilled, can burn the skin • may be fatal if swallowed • mixing Viagra with alkyl nitrites may increase the risk of heart problems	• amyl nitrite is a prescription-only medicine • possession is not illegal, but supply can be an offence
AMPHETAMINES	speed, whizz, uppers, amph, billy, sulphate	• grey or white powder that is snorted, swallowed, smoked, injected or dissolved in a drink • tablets which are swallowed	• excitement – the mind races and users feel confident and energetic	• while on the drug, some users become tense and anxious • leaves users feeling tired and depressed for one or two days and sometimes longer • high doses repeated over a few days may cause panic and hallucinations • long-term use puts a strain on the heart • heavy, long-term use can lead to mental illness • mixing Viagra with amphetamines may increase the risk of heart problems	class B (but class A if prepared for injection)
CANNABIS	marijuana, draw, blow, weed, puff, shit, hash, ganja, spliff, wacky backy **Cannabis is the most commonly used drug among 11 to 25 year olds**	• a solid, dark lump known as 'resin' • leaves, stalks and seeds called 'grass' • a sticky, dark oil • can be rolled (usually with tobacco) in a spliff or joint, smoked on its own in a special pipe, or cooked and eaten in food	• users feel relaxed and talkative • cooking the drug then eating it makes the effects more intense and harder to control • may bring on a craving for food (this is often referred to as having the 'munchies')	• smoking it with tobacco may lead to users becoming hooked on cigarettes • impairs the ability to learn and concentrate • can leave people tired and lacking energy • users may lack motivation and feel apathetic • can make users paranoid and anxious, depending on their mood and situation • smoking joints over a long period of time can lead to respiratory disorders, including lung cancer	class B (but class A penalties can apply to cannabis oil)

ECSTASY	E, doves, XTC, disco biscuits, echoes, hug drug, burgers, fantasy chemical name: MDMA (currently many tablets contain MDEA, MDA, MBDB) **4% of 16 to 25s have used ecstasy in the last 3 months**	tablets of different shapes, size and colour (but often white) which are swallowed	• users feel alert and in tune with their surroundings • sound, colour and emotions seem much more intense • users may dance for hours • the effects last from 3 to 6 hours	• can leave users feeling tired and depressed for days • risk of overheating and dehydration if users dance energetically without taking breaks or drinking enough fluids (users should sip about a pint of non-alcoholic fluid such as fruit juice, sports drinks or water every hour) • use has been linked to liver and kidney problems • some experts are concerned that use of ecstasy can lead to brain damage causing depression in later life • mixing Viagra with ecstasy may increase the risk of heart problems	class A other drugs similar to ecstasy are also illegal and class A
GASES, GLUES & AEROSOLS	products such as lighter gas refills, aerosols containing products such as hairspray, deodorants and air fresheners, tins or tubes of glue, some paints, thinners and correcting fluids	• sniffed or breathed into the lungs from a cloth or sleeve • gas products are sometimes squirted directly into the back of the throat	• effects feel similar to being very drunk • users feel thick-headed, dizzy, giggly and dreamy • users may hallucinate • effects don't last very long, but users can remain intoxicated all day by repeating the dose	• nausea, vomiting, black-outs and heart problems that can be fatal • squirting gas products down the throat may cause the body to produce fluid that floods the lungs and this can cause instant death • risk of suffocation if the substance is inhaled from a plastic bag over the head • accidents can happen when the user is high because their senses are affected • long-term abuse of glue can damage the brain, liver and kidneys	it is illegal for shopkeepers to sell to under-18s, or to people acting for them, if they suspect the product is intended for abuse

	other names include	what it looks like & how it is taken	the effects	the health risks	legal status
HEROIN	smack, brown, horse, gear, junk, H, jack, scag	brownish-white powder which is smoked, snorted or dissolved and injected	• small doses give the user a sense of warmth and well-being • larger doses can make them drowsy and relaxed	• heroin is addictive (even when smoked) • users who form a habit may end up taking the drug just to feel normal • excessive amounts can result in overdose, coma and in some cases death • injecting can damage veins • sharing injecting equipment puts users at risk of dangerous infections like hepatitis B or C and HIV/AIDS	class A
LSD	acid, trips, tabs, blotters, microdots, dots	¹/₄ inch squares of paper, often with a picture on one side, which are swallowed. Microdots and dots are tiny tablets	• effects are known as a 'trip' and can last for 8 to 12 hours • users will experience their surroundings in a very different way • sense of movement and time may speed up or slow down • objects, colours and sounds may be distorted	• once a trip starts it cannot be stopped • users may have a 'bad trip', which can be terrifying • 'flashbacks' may be experienced where parts of a trip are re-lived some time after the event • can complicate mental health problems	class A

For more information about these or any other drugs   call the National Drugs Helpline on 0800 77 66 00

TABLE 2.4 *Illegal drugs*

Almost one in six young people takes illegal drugs on a regular basis, according to a recent survey, and almost half of all young people have taken drugs at sometime in their life. The survey showed that men aged between 156 and 29 who drink and smoke heavily, are unemployed, and go out a lot in the evenings are most likely to take illegal drugs.

It can be very difficult to tell if a person is using drugs. Signs that parents are encouraged to look out for include the following:

- Sudden changes of mood from happy to alert to sullen and moody;
- Unusual irritability or aggression;
- Loss of appetite;
- Loss of interest in hobbies, sport, school work or friends;
- Bouts of drowsiness or sleepiness;
- Increased evidence of telling lies or furtive behaviour;
- Unexplained loss of money or belongings from the home;
- Unusual smells, stains, or marks on the body or clothes, or around the house.

(NB. Some of these signs are a normal part of growing up, and it is important that people do not jump to conclusions).

It is difficult to describe the exact effects of a drug because the effect is influenced by:

- the amount taken
- how much the user has taken before
- what the user wants and expects to happen
- the surroundings in which it is taken
- the reactions of other people

A person who feels they need to keep taking a drug, is known as 'drug dependent'. This dependence may be either **physical** or **psychological**.

Physical dependence: Withdrawal from the drug involves physical discomfort.

Psychological dependence: Withdrawal from the drug results in craving or emotional distress. This is the most widespread and important type of dependence.

Illegal drug use can be particularly harmful to a developing foetus. The unborn baby can be harmed by:

- Drug use affecting the mother's health either directly or through self–neglect and poor nutrition;
- Drugs may directly affect the foetus through the mother's blood stream. There are particular risks associated with the injection of drugs;

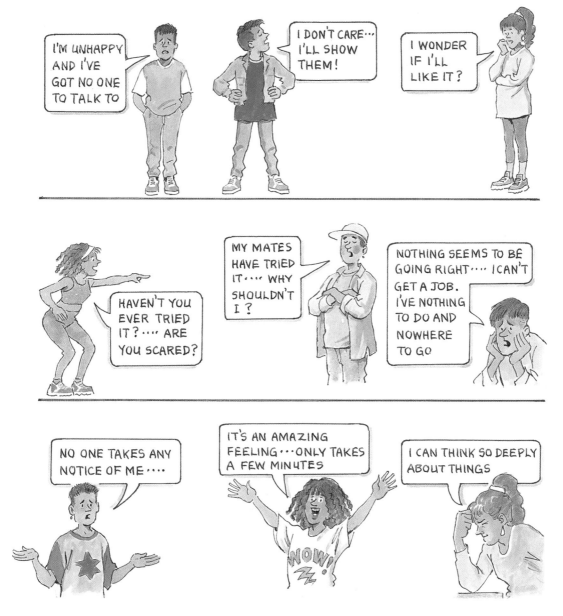

FIGURE 2.18 *Why do people take drugs?*

- Infection may result from the use of non–sterile needles. (For example, the transmission of HIV or hepatitis);
- Abscesses and gangrene may be caused by missing the vein when injecting;

Figure 2.18 shows some of the reasons for drug taking.

There is a wide variety of help available for people with drug problems. Details of the services available can be obtained from the National Drugs Helpline (see References and Resources section at the end of the chapter.) These services are provided by the NHS and voluntary organisations and can link in with other services such as social care, housing or legal advice. The type of help available includes:

- Information about drugs;
- Support for drug users and their families;
- Out patient clinics for treating drug users (E.g. The prescription of illegal drug substitutes);
- In patient treatment for more serious complications;
- Residential rehabilitation services to help people recover from their dependency.

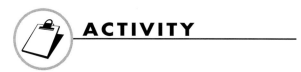

ACTIVITY

1 **What advice would you give to a parent who finds out that their child is using illegal drugs?**
2 **Find out what to do if you were to find someone very drowsy or unconscious because of drug taking (see end of Chapter for answers.)**
3 **Look at Table 2.4 which lists a number of illegal drugs. Discuss which age groups are most likely to use each drug.**

Use and abuse of legal drugs

There are a number of drugs which are used legally. When their use is considered harmful or socially unacceptable, this is considered to be **abuse**. Far more deaths are caused each year through the abuse of legal drugs than from illegal drugs. The commonest legally used drugs are:

- Caffeine
- Alcohol
- Nicotine

CAFFEINE

Caffeine is the most widely used drug in the world. It is a stimulant which is found in coffee, tea, chocolate and cola drinks. Caffeine produces physical dependence, and in high doses (for example, six cups of strong coffee a day) can cause harmful effects. However, caffeine may not be all bad. Unlike alcohol and nicotine, it does not kill and can improve athletic performance. It is sometimes used to treat weak breathing in premature babies.

I walked into the smoke-filled room and breathed a sigh of relief. It was obvious I could get what I was looking for. Scoring is never very difficult in a place like this and it was obvious that I could not only get my drug of choice, but I could get it in any combination I desired. The dealers were polite enough, and even offered to bring it over to the table. I remember the first time I had indulged. It used to make me sick, but over the years I had built up a tolerance. Anyway, this was a drug I could handle; it made me feel better, more sociable; gave me a bit of a glow.'

(From: "Booze: Britain's real drug crisis' in The Independent 7.8.98.)

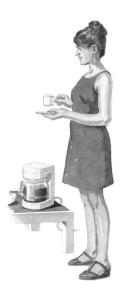

FIGURE 2.19 *Harmful effects of caffeine*

Reading the account above, you probably thought an illegal drug was being described, but this is an account of obtaining the legal drug, alcohol. However, because a drug is legal it must not be considered harmless.

- There are an estimated 5000 deaths each year in England and Wales directly related to alcohol. (For heroin there are about 350 deaths in a year, and for ecstasy, fewer than 10).
- Deaths from alcohol–related diseases have increased by more than a third in the past 10 years.
- One in 20 people are addicted to alcohol.
- About 27% of adult males drink above the level recommended by the medical profession.
- Alcohol costs the NHS £1.5 million a year.
- Alcohol costs British industry an estimated £2 billion a year due to absenteeism and poor performance.
- Alcohol is a factor in 40% of domestic violence.

Young people and alcohol

- In 1997 1000 children under 15 were admitted to hospital suffering from acute alcohol poisoning.
- In the past 10 years 55 teenagers have died after drinking too much alcohol.
- Three quarters of all 11 year olds have tried alcohol.
- The average weekly amount of alcohol consumed by 11–15 year olds doubled between 1990 and 1996.
- 1000 children aged under 15 are admitted to hospital each year with acute alcohol poisoning.
- Young people who regularly use alcohol are 22 times more likely to go on to use illegal drugs.
- Children of alcoholics have a greater risk of becoming alcoholics themselves.

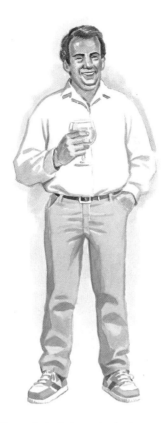

FIGURE 2.20 *The long term affects of alcohol on the body.*

What can parents do to help? The Health Education Authority give the advice to parents that they should not try to prevent children from drinking and then drink too much themselves. They should talk about alcohol when they are young and teach them that drinking in moderation is acceptable, but binge drinking can be very dangerous.

Pregnancy and alcohol

Alcohol can stop the normal development of the foetus. Babies born to mothers who drink large amounts of alcohol throughout the pregnancy may be born with **foetal alcohol syndrome**. These children have facial deformities, stunted growth and mental retardation. More moderate drinking may increase the risk of miscarriage, but many women continue to drink small amounts of alcohol throughout their pregnancy with no ill effects. Pregnant women are recommended to have no more than one or two alcoholic drinks a week. The same advice is given to women who are breastfeeding.

The elderly and alcohol

- At least a third of elderly drinkers did not have a problem with alcohol until they reached the age of 60.
- Older people are at greater risk of alcohol related issues such as hypothermia, incontinence and depression.

- Elderly alcoholics suffer more severe withdrawal symptoms than younger people.
- Elders use the most prescription drugs, and alcohol can cause serious side effects when combined with many of these.

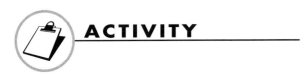

ACTIVITY

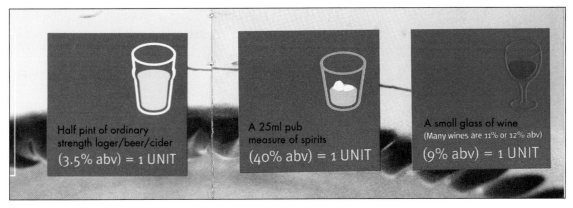

FIGURE 2.21 *Drinks containing 1 unit of alcohol*

Taken from "Think About Drink" Health Education Authority leaflet

1 **One of the most important things for drinkers to know is how the alcohol content of different drinks compare. Figure 2.21 shows drinks which contain roughly the same amount of alcohol. Each of these can be thought of as a unit. Table 2.5 shows the limits people should keep below to avoid damaging their health.**

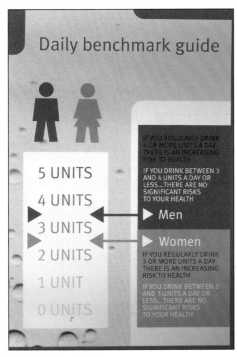

TABLE 2.5 *Limits to drinking to prevent damage to health.*

Copy out Table 2.6 to help you keep a diary of your alcohol consumption for a typical week (or if more appropriate ask an adult to do this for you.). At the end of the week calculate the number of units consumed. Compare this with the recommended limits. If the amount consumed is high, identify suitable opportunities for cutting down. (It is sometimes worth remembering HALT. This is to remind people that the occasions when there is the greatest temptation to drink too much are when someone is hungry, angry, lonely or tired.)

Drink Diary

	What?	Where / when / who with	Units
Mon			
Tues			
Wed			
Thur			
Fri			
Sat			
Sun			
		TOTAL :	

TABLE 2.6 *Drink diary*

2 'When a teenager dies after taking Ecstasy it's front page news. The Government now warns us of a new heroin epidemic. But a far more deadly and acceptable substance is freely available at a bar, restaurant or supermarket near you – Booze: Britain's real drug crisis'

The headline above appeared recently in a national newspaper (The Independent 7.8.98). In what ways do you think alcohol can be considered 'Britain's real drug crisis'?

3 The following measures have been suggested to help limit the problems caused by excess drinking:

- The drink drive limits should be lowered
- More alcohol education should be provided for young people
- Bottles and cans should carry the number of units in a bottle or can
- Better services should be provided to people addicted to alcohol

Discuss how successful you think each of these measures would be.

NICOTINE

Smoking is the biggest single cause of preventable disease and premature death. There are five times more people killed by smoking than by road accident, suicide, murder, AIDS, and illegal drugs put together.

Nicotine is the powerful drug in tobacco which causes physical and psychological addiction to smoking. It increases heart rate and blood pressure.

Other things in cigarette smoke which cause harm are:

Tar
This is black and sticky and contains cancer causing chemicals (carcinogens). Tar clogs up the lungs and the chemicals are gradually absorbed, causing irritation and damage.

Carbon monoxide
This is a harmful gas which makes blood less efficient at carrying oxygen to the brain and muscles.

Young people and smoking
The longer someone smokes, the greater their chance of serious health problems later on. Because nicotine is addictive, the earlier someone starts smoking the harder it is for them to give up in later life.

Trying out new things and taking risks is a part of growing up, and figures show that 60% of all 15 year olds have smoked. Children are twice as likely to smoke if their parents are regular smokers.

Pregnancy, parenthood and smoking
A pregnant woman who smokes:

- is more likely to have an underweight baby
- twice as likely to have a premature baby
- a third more likely to have a stillborn baby
- more likely to have a miscarriage

Children who have a parent who smokes:

- are at a higher risk of cot death
- are a third more likely to suffer from glue ear which causes partial deafness
- are twice as likely to suffer from chest infections
- are twice as likely to have asthma attacks

It is therefore important that as well as giving up smoking for the duration of the pregnancy, parents should make every effort not to smoke in the company of their young children.

The elderly and smoking
Studies have shown that smokers aged 65 to 74 years old are almost 10 times more likely to die of lung cancer than those of this age group who do not smoke. Because of the harmful effects of continuing to smoke, even in old age, it is important that elderly people consider trying to stop. However, this may be more difficult for them because the longer a person has smoked for, the stronger the addiction to nicotine.

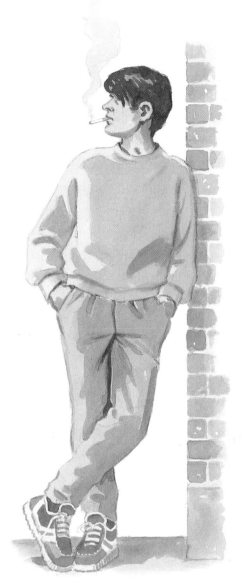

FIGURE 2.22 *Smoking is the biggest single cause of preventable disease.*

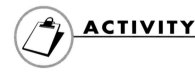 **ACTIVITY**

1   Make a poster, leaflet, or booklet aimed at encouraging a person to give up smoking. Aim it at either:

   ● a young person
   ● a pregnant woman
   ● a parent of a young child
   ● an elderly person

2   Find out about the Nicotine Replacement Therapies on offer – patches, gums and inhalers. How much do they cost, how are they used, and, if you have the opportunity to talk to users, how successful are they?

DIETS WHICH PUT HEALTH AT RISK

If a person's diet is not balanced, and has an excess or inadequate amount of particular nutrients, their health will suffer. In developing countries the most common causes of malnutrition are lack of protein and energy in the diet, but in developed countries unhealthy diets tend to include too much salt, sugar, and fatty foods which are linked to cancer, heart disease, stroke and tooth decay.

Obesity

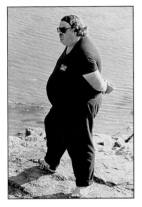

FIGURE 2.23 *In recent years there has been an increase in the number of people classified as obese.*

Obesity or fatness runs in families and results from taking in more energy from the diet than is used up by the body. This is likely to happen if a person has a high sugar and/or fat diet.

Obesity can lead to emotional and social problems, as well as physical problems such as an increased likelihood of suffering from heart problems, high blood pressure, cancer of the colon, and diabetes. In the UK in 1995, about 4% of children were considered to be obese, and obese children are likely to become obese adults (Figure 2.23).

Anorexia Nervosa

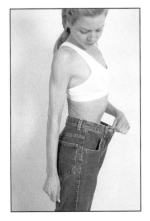

FIGURE 2.24 *A person suffering from Anorexia.*

Anorexia is often, but wrongly, known as the 'slimmer's disease'. It mainly affects adolescent girls, although it can affect children from as young as seven to people in middle age, and males as well as females can be affected (Figure 2.24).

People with anorexia are likely to show the following characteristics:

● Extreme weight loss
● Over activity and excessive exercising
● Tiredness and weakness
● Lanugo (baby–like hair on the body, thinning of hair on head)
● Extreme choosiness over food

There are various theories over what causes the illness. For example:

● Those affected by anorexia see it as a way of taking control over their lives.
● Affected individuals do not wish to grow up and are trying to keep their childhood shape. This may partly result from the media obsession with achieving the 'perfect' (i.e. slim) body
● It may be a physical illness caused partly by hormonal changes
● It may be caused by depression

Bulimia nervosa

Bulimia nervosa is characterised by episodes of compulsive overeating usually followed by self–induced vomiting. Again, the majority of individuals affected are female.

People with the disorder are likely to show the following characteristics:

● The affected individual may be of normal weight, or only slightly underweight
● Bingeing or vomiting may occur once or several times a day
● The individual may have depression
● The acid present in the vomit may damage teeth enamel
● As with anorexia, there is no single cause to account for the disorder

Girls suffering 'unhealthy obsession' with slimming/ Home News
JOHN CARVEL

GIRLS in their mid-teens are developing an unhealthy obsession with slimming and nearly half have the mistaken impression they are overweight, according to a survey published yesterday by the Schools Health Education Unit.

At the ages of 14 and 15, one in five have nothing for breakfast and another 19 per cent take only a drink before leaving for school. One in seven do not eat lunch.

But the results coincide with an unrealistic view among the same group of girls about how much they needed to diet. Six out of 10 thought they needed to lose weight, even though only 15.3 per cent did weigh too much for their age and height.

Boys of the same age had a more realistic attitude. Just over a quarter said they would like to lose weight, while just under one in five were actually overweight.

The boys said they drank more fizzy drinks and at more chips than the girls. About half the girls ate salads at least two days a week. Among both groups, low fat milk was more popular than ordinary milk.

The British Dietetic Association said that the survey raised serious concerns about the health of teenage girls. "From these figures, it would seem that the problem of girls skimping meals to lose weight is getting worse." said Lyndel Costain, its spokeswoman.

Only 1 to 2 per cent of girls developed severe eating disorders such as bulimia and anorexia, compared with the 60-70 per cent who dieted. "But there is a bigger group of girls who may nevertheless be putting their health at risk by skimping meals in this way."

"Girls of 14 and 15 are still growing and need things like iron and calcium to ensure that they grow up healthy. Girls with eating patterns like these may not develop anorexia, but they may nevertheless be doing themselves psychological or physical harm." she said.

18 March 1998, The Guardian, p.8

Food Giants want you to carry on eating salt – even if it kills you

by Marie Woolf and John Illman

The food industry is fighting a rearguard action to keep Britons on a high-salt diet – although it can cause high blood pressure and head to strokes, heart attacks and kidney failure.

High salt intake has been linked to stomach cancer and there is growing evidence that it could cause loss of calcium and be a major factor in osteoporosis (thinning of bones).

About 80 per cent of the salt Britons eat is hidden in processed foods, some of which contain as much salt as sea-water. The Committee of Medical Aspects of Food recently warned that we should eat no more than six grams of salt a day (about one level teaspoon), yet the average adult has nine grams.

The food industry claims salt is needed because it acts as a flavour enhancer, preservative and processing aid.

The present government has to decide whether to bow to pressure from the industry or issue guidance on cutting down on salt. 'Salt should be the number one nutrition priority' said Jack Winkler, a food policy analyst.

The Observer 7 June 1998

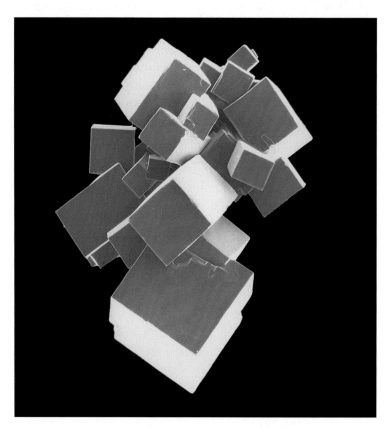

FIGURE 2.25 *A photograph of common salt (sodium chloride) crystals viewed with an electron microscope.*

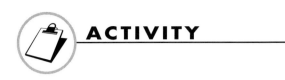

ACTIVITY

1 (i) Collect photographs from magazines of models wearing clothes which are likely to appeal to young women. Do the models look healthy? Do you think that the body shape of these models is likely to influence adolescent girls?

   (ii) 'Teenage dolls (such as Cindy and Barbie) promote an idealised role model which is unhealthy and can damage the self–concept of the child.' Discuss what this statement means, and whether you agree with it.

2 Read the article 'Girls suffering 'unhealthy obsession' with slimming'. If you have the opportunity, carry out your own survey of boys and girls between the ages of nine and sixteen to find out:

   i)   How many eat breakfast;

   ii)   How many eat lunch;

   iii) How many think they need to lose weight

   (Express your answers as percentages and draw a bar graph to compare the results for boys and girls.)

3 Read the newspaper article on salt in the diet, and answer the following questions:

   i)   List the diseases a high salt diet is thought to cause

   ii)   In which foods is most of the salt in our diet found?

   iii) What is recommended as the maximum amount of salt we should have in our diet?

   iv)   What do the food industry say we need salt for?

Stress

If there is a change in a person's life, which they find difficult to cope with, we say they are suffering from stress.

ACTIVITY

1 Factors which cause stress are known as *stressors*. Examples of stressors are:

   ● bereavement

   ● the birth of a child

   ● moving house

   Can you think of examples of other stressors?

2 Doctors sometimes classify people as Type A or Type B. Read the characteristics below and decide which type best describes you.

CHARACTERISTICS OF TYPE A:	CHARACTERISTICS OF TYPE B:
Hardworking	Easy going manner
A lot of drive	Relaxed
Enjoy a challenge	Calm
Feel guilty when relaxing	Non–aggressive
Uneasy if not 'on the go'	Tolerant
Competitive	
Ambitious	

Type A people are more likely to suffer from stress. For example, they are twice as likely to develop coronary heart disease.

If a person is under excessive stress, they will perform a task poorly. However, stress should not always be thought of as entirely negative. If a person is completely lacking stress, to the point at which they are bored, there will also be a decline in their ability to perform a task (Fig. 2.26). This means that for each person there will be an optimum level of stress which will help them perform to the best of their ability.

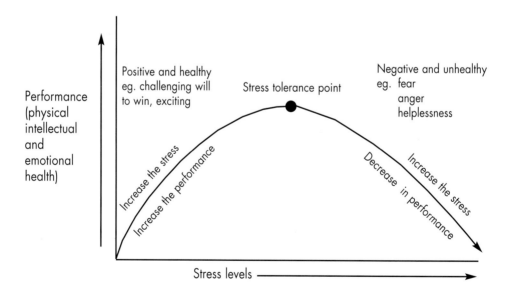

FIGURE 2.26 *The relationship; between amount of stress and the ability to perform a task.*

Stress and how we manage our stress levels is linked directly to our health. A constant unmanageable level of stress will lead to physical, emotional and intellectual ill health.

When a person is under stress, the hormone adrenaline is produced. This hormone prepares you for what is known as the 'alarm' or 'fight or flight' reaction.

Some of the effects of adrenaline include:

- an increased heart rate
- less blood flowing through the skin, which may make a person appear pale
- less blood flowing around the gut, which leads to the feeling of 'butterflies'
- increased sweating.

If the stress continues, eventually the adrenal gland, which produces adrenaline, will no longer function properly and the person will become ill. More than a quarter of a million British people are absent from work each day because of stress related illnesses, and it is estimated that these cost £7 billion per year in sick pay, lost production and health service provision.

There are various disorders which are triggered by stress. For example:

- *Physical health problems*, such as stomach ulcers, heart attacks, skin disorders such as eczema and psoriasis, myalgic encephalomyelitis (ME).
- *Emotional effects*, such as anxiety, insomnia and depression.
- *Behavioural effects*, such as increased smoking or consumption of alcohol. Table 2.7 shows many of the short term and long term symptoms of stress.

BEHAVIOURAL SHORT TERM	PHYSICAL SHORT TERM	EMOTIONAL SHORT TERM
Over indulgence in smoking, alcohol or drugs	Headaches	Tiredness
Accidents	Back aches	Anxiety
Impulsive, emotional behaviour	Sleeping badly	Boredom
Poor relationships with others at home and at work	Indigestion	Irritability
Poor work performance	nausea	Depression
Emotional withdrawal	Dizziness	Inability to concentrate
	Excessive sweating	Apathy
	Trembling	

BEHAVIOURAL LONG TERM	PHYSICAL LONG TERM	EMOTIONAL LONG TERM
Marital and family breakdown	Heart disease	Insomnia
Social isolation	Hypertension	Chronic depression and anxiety
	Ulcers	
	Poor general health	

TABLE 2.7 *Symptoms of stress.*

"Stress at Work" Health and Safety leaflet. Published by UNISON

Methods of coping with stressful situations may be either beneficial to a person's health or harmful to their health. For example, if you have an examination in a week on a topic you find difficult, you may choose any of the following methods to help you cope:

Methods of coping which are beneficial to health:

➡ **Changing work patterns**. For example, you could draw up a revision timetable which allows you to spend an hour going through the work each evening with a friend.

➡ **Exercise**. For example, you could make time to go for an early morning swim.

➡ The use of relaxation techniques. For example, you could attend a yoga class.

➡ **A healthy diet**. You should make time to enjoy healthy, well–balanced meals.

➡ **An increase in leisure time**. For example, you could spend time at the weekend relaxing with friends.

➡ **Rest**. You should make sure you have at least 6 – 8 hours sleep a night.

Methods of coping which are harmful to health:

➡ Increased use of tobacco, alcohol, tranquillisers, sleeping pills or illegal drugs.

➡ Long hours of studying causing lack of sleep.

 ACTIVITY

1 Interview a student to find out how they cope with stressful situations related to their studies, for example, important assignment deadlines or unit tests. Identify which of their methods of copying may be harmful to their health, and suggest more beneficial alternatives.

2 List the things that cause you stress. For example, waiting for a bus, sitting in a traffic jam, working on a difficult assignment, giving an oral presentation. Once you have identified the things that cause you stress, consciously try to relax in these situations and, where possible, do what you can to tackle the source of the problem. For example, before giving an oral presentation, make sure you are really well prepared, breathe in and then breathe out slowly a few times before starting, and consciously relax your shoulders.

Personal Hygiene

A dictionary definition of hygiene is *'The science concerned with maintenance of health'*. However, we usually think of hygiene as being concerned with preventing pathogens entering the body. Pathogens are disease–causing organisms, mainly bacteria and viruses. These can enter the body through:

● the skin (for example, through cuts, sweat pores and hair follicles)

● the alimentary canal (gut)

● the respiratory tract (throat, trachea and lungs)

To maintain high levels of hygiene we need the following:

- Efficient sewage disposal
- Clean water supply
- Efficient refuse disposal
- Clean air (for example, good room ventilation)
- Good personal hygiene (for example, care of teeth, hair and skin)
- Safe food handling and preparation

 ACTIVITY

Choose one of the six precautions necessary for good hygiene which are listed above and prepare a poster to explain how it should be carried out. If you are working in a group, try to ensure that all six topics are covered.

Lack of Exercise

As the section on exercise above (pages 172–176) explained, physical activity is important for all aspects of our health.

 ACTIVITY

Read the news paper article below (Times 18.6.98).
- If possible talk to at least one 11 – 15 year old who does not walk to school, and find out their reasons for this.
- What steps are being taken in your neighbourhood to encourage children to walk to school?

Fears for health as children walk less

The growing trend of driving children to and from school has contributed to a marked decline in walking by teenagers, according to a government report. The rate at which the number of walks taken by those aged between 11 and 15 is falling is more than twice that for the population as a whole. The statistics have prompted fears that the health of teenagers will suffer.

Over the ten years to 1996, the 11-15 age group reduced their number of walks by 29 per cent, against 13 per cent for other age groups. The government survey shows the average person making 22 fewer journeys a year on foot but an extra 203 journeys by car.

Source: The Times 18/6/98

Sexual Behaviour

In the 1980's in response to the discovery of AIDS, there were a number of prominent advertising campaigns alerting the public to the danger of 'unsafe sex' (i.e. sexual intercourse without the use of a condom).

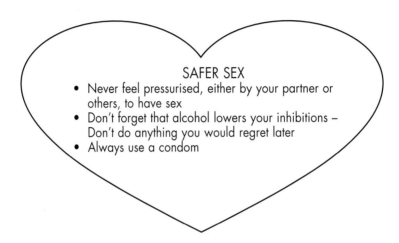

SAFER SEX
- Never feel pressurised, either by your partner or others, to have sex
- Don't forget that alcohol lowers your inhibitions – Don't do anything you would regret later
- Always use a condom

FIGURE 2.27 *Advice given by the Health Education Authority on Safer Sex.*

As well as helping to control the spread of HIV, this also had the effect of limiting the number of cases of other sexually transmitted diseases (STD's). However, now people are apparently becoming more complacent about the need to practice safe sex, according to a recent survey. It found that the number of 18 to 20 year olds having unprotected sex had doubled in the past year. This helps to explain why the level of STD's is increasing again and why Britain has the highest teenage birth rate in Western Europe. Look at Figure 2.27 for advice given by The Health Education Authority on Safer Sex.

Table 2.8 lists some of the common STD's.

Genital herpes (HSV) is caused by the herpes simplex virus. It can be passed on through skin contact with an infected person through kissing, penetrative sex or oral sex. It can affect the mouth, the genital area, the skin around the anus and the fingers in the form of blisters and sores, sometimes accompanied by flu-like symptoms. After the initial outbreak is over the virus hides away in the nerve fibres, where it remains totally undetected and causes no symptoms. It can recur when the person is ill or run down, but is not so severe in its symptoms. Treatment is usually unnecessary but tablets are available to reduce the severity of symptoms when it is first caught, if treated quickly.

Gonorrhoea is a bacterial infection. It is sexually transmitted and can infect the cervix, urethra, rectum, anus and throat. It sometimes causes no symptoms but can include discharge from the penis in men and vagina in women (including pain when urinating), and from the anus in both sexes. Treatment is administered through antibiotics. It is important for both sexes to receive treatment but women should be aware that it can lead to infertility if left untreated.

Chlamydia is the most common treatable bacterial sexually transmitted infection. It infects the cervix in women, and can infect the urethra, rectum and eyes in both sexes, causing discharge from the genitals, pain when passing urine, swollen eyes and other symptoms. Women should be checked if their sexual partner displays these symptoms, even if they experience no symptoms themselves, as it can lead to infertility. Treatment is administered through antibiotics.

Genital warts are small fleshy growths which may appear anywhere on a man or woman's genital area. They are caused by the human papilloma virus (HPV) and are passed on through genital contact. They are treated by liquid solutions, by freezing or by lasers, but may need prolonged treatment before they disappear. It is also possible that they will recur so further check ups at a clinic of genito-urinary medicine (GUM) will be necessary. Treatment is important as some types of the wart virus may be linked to changes in cervical cells which can lead to cervical cancer in women.

HIV (Human Immunodeficiency Virus) is a virus that can damage the body's defence system so that it cannot fight off certain infections. If someone with HIV goes on to get certain serious illnesses, this condition is called AIDS. The virus is passed on through unprotected vaginal or anal sex with someone who has HIV, by sharing needles, syringes or other drug-injecting equipment with someone who has HIV, or from a mother with HIV to her baby during pregnancy, at birth or during breastfeeding. Thee are no early warning symptoms of the virus and at present there is no cure or vaccine. There are, however, new drugs that can control the level of HIV in the blood and delay the development of AIDS. HIV can be avoided by practising safe sex (any sex that does not allow blood, semen or fluid from the vagina to be exchanged internally, e.g. get inside the body) and by avoiding the sharing of needles when injecting drugs.

TABLE 2.8 *Some of the common STD's*

A person with an STD may have no symptoms, or they may have leakage from the penis or vagina, rashes, itchiness, sores, blisters, pain in the genital region, or a burning sensation when urinating or having sex. Most STD's can be treated quickly and easily, but some can cause long term problems if untreated. It is, therefore, essential that anyone who is worried that they may have contacted an STD goes to the Doctor or special clinics as soon as possible. The name of these clinics varies from one part of the country to another. It could be called Genito-Urinary Medicine (GUM) Clinic, Sexually Transmitted Disease Clinic, Venereal Disease (VD) Clinic, or Sexual Health Clinic. These treat everyone in confidence.

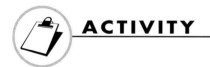 **ACTIVITY**

Have a go at the following quiz (See end of Chapter for Answers.)

1 **Sexually transmitted diseases can cause:**
   a)   **itchiness and a burning sensation when urinating**
   b)   **infertility if untreated**
   c)   **no symptoms**
   d)   **all of the above**

2 To be effective, emergency contraceptive pills must be taken:
   a) the morning after having unprotected sex
   b) up to 3 days after having unprotected sex
   c) up to a week after having unprotected sex

3 HIV can be passed on by which of the following:
   a) kissing
   b) toilet seats
   c) towels
   d) sheets
   e) cups
   f) swimming pools
   g) unprotected sex

Unsafe Practices in the Work Place

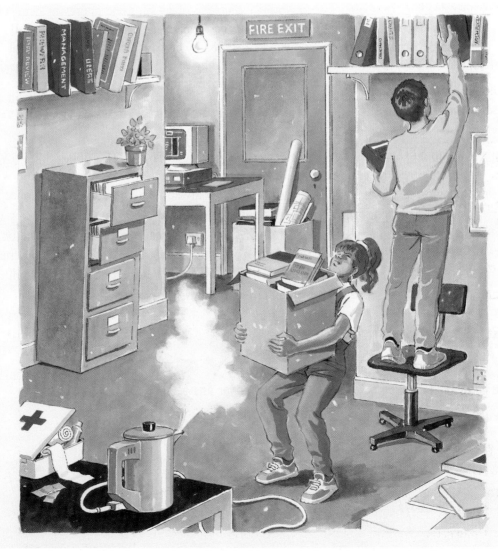

FIGURE 2.28 *Unsafe practices in the work place – how many hazards can you identify?*
(See end of Chapter for Answers.)

There are 1000,000 major injuries caused by accidents at work every year, including 600 deaths. By law, all employers and employees should be aware of health and safety matters. Each industry has safety standards that must be met. These are drawn up by advisory committees which consider the following areas:

1 Major hazards
2 Toxic substances
3 Dangerous substances
4 Medical
5 Nuclear safety
6 Dangerous pathogens
7 Industrial — paper, oil, agriculture, Health Services, printing, foundries, construction, railway.

If the employer is negligent, they may have to pay fines and compensation to the victims of accidents, or even face imprisonment. However, it must also be remembered that the personal responsibility of employees is very important.

There are certain conditions which are classed as **occupational disorders** because they are caused by hazards at work. These include:

● Dust diseases (These are caused by inhaling dust, for example, in mining.)
● Chemical poisoning.
● Noise damage.
● Radiation damage. (This may affect people working in outdoor occupations in sunny climates or people working in the nuclear industry).
● Repetitive strain injury. (Pain in joints and muscles caused by repeated movement of part of the body.)

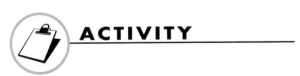

ACTIVITY

1 **List the potential hazards at work that may affect people in the following professions:**
    ● **nursing**
    ● **science teaching**
    ● **social work**
    ● **building work**
    If possible check your list with people employed in these professions.
2 **An investigation — health and safety at work in your school or college**
    Produce a report called 'Potential Safety Hazards in the College/School'.
    ● **In pairs, make a general survey of the health and safety facilities and considerations throughout the establishment. (You may prefer to concentrate on just one particular area or department.) Make a note of safety equipment, for example fire escapes, fire drill instructions and first aid facilities.,**

- Any employers who employ more than five people have a legal duty to provide a written health and safety policy. Ask to see a copy of this.
- Make notes on possible hazards such as dangerous equipment and furniture. Use photographs and diagrams to illustrate your report.
- Interview staff and students to find out about any Health and Safety problems and solutions. Tape your interviews.
- In pairs, give a presentation to your class.

3 Look at Figure 2.28. Identify all the unsafe practices you can see in this work place.

....

Health Promotion

Health Promotion is one of the most important aspects of this unit. There are a number of different definitions of health promotion, but one which is often used is the WHO (World Health Organisation) definition:

"Health promotion is the process of enabling people to increase control over, and to improve, their health."

Health promotion involves providing information to others which will help them to improve their health and well–being. It may also include the development of **health improvement plans**, either for groups or individuals.

Stages in the development of a health improvement plan:

1 The **health risks** of a person, or group, must be identified from:
   - **data relating to measures of health**, for example, blood pressure or pulse rate data (See section on 'Indicators of good physical health' on page 211 below),
   - **lifestyle information**
2 **Aims** and **objectives** must be set. What health improvements (targets) are we aiming for?
3 **Methods** and **activities** must be planned. How are we going to bring about the hoped for health improvements?
4 **Resources** must be identified. Which organisations, books, leaflets, posters, advertisements, websites etc. will provide useful information? (See section on 'Resources' at the end of the chapter.)
5 The health improvement plan is **implemented**.
6 The success of the health plan must be **evaluated**. Have the targets been met? If not, why not? What improvements could be made?

Some of the features of a successful health plan:

- As much information as possible must be gathered on **lifestyle** and **physical indicators of good health** (eg. height:weight ratio) to allow the risks of an individual or a group to be identified.
- The plan should consider **physical, social** and **emotional** health.

- The person putting the plan together have **empathy** for the feelings of the person for whom the plan has been created, and understand that a person's choice about their health and well-being can be affected by self-esteem, financial factors and social pressures.

- The plan should include **short- and long-term targets** with time-scales. For example, a short-term target could be to increase physical activity which in the long-term would improve levels of fitness.

- Targets should be **realistic**. For example, a very rapid weight loss may be considered unrealistic.

- The **strengths** and **weaknesses** of the plan should be identified. It is important to remember that activities to improve health, such as dieting and increasing exercise, involve determination from the person following the plan. It is likely that some parts of the plan will be more challenging to achieve than other parts and these should be anticipated with suggestions made of how to overcome difficulties.

- The plan, including the language used, should **reflect the needs and abilities of the chosen target**, for example, child, adolescent, adult, or elderly person.

- Relevant **health promotional material** should be identified and used appropriately. (See 'Useful Resources' section at the end of the chapter.)

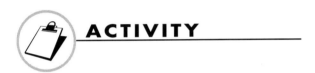

ACTIVITY

1   The website www.HealthCentral.com allows you to crate a health profile by answering a number of questions on your life style. It then identifies your greatest health risks and gives you advice on changes you could make to improve your health. Have a go!

2   At the end of this chapter there are a number of opportunities for you to prepare and develop health plans. One of these can be used as your portfolio work for grading which will give you a grade for this unit.

....

Indicators of Physical Good Health

There are many factors that can be measured in order to help make an assessment of someone's physical health.

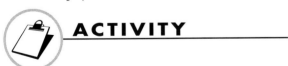

ACTIVITY

Have you ever been for a medical, for example when starting a new school or job? (If not try to find someone who has and question them.) What measurements were made?

....

The following list gives examples of measurements that may be taken in an assessment of a person's physical health:

● Height
● Weight
● Pulse rate (at rest/after exercise)
● Blood pressure
● Lung capacity

In this unit you need to know how the following can be used to measure good health:

● Height and Weight
● Body mass index
● Peak flow
● Resting pulse rate and recovery after exercise.

HEIGHT AND WEIGHT

A person's weight can be an important guide to their physical health. If someone was very overweight or underweight it would obviously give cause for concern about their physical health. However, as the example below shows, a measurement of weight alone will not give sufficient information to allow conclusions to be reached about physical fitness.

 ACTIVITY

Paul is an 18 year old student who weighs 77kg. Can you make any comments on the state of his physical health?

What other piece of information would be most useful to help you form an opinion?

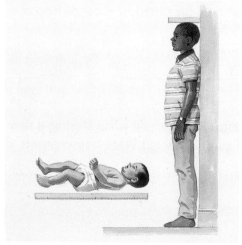

FIGURE 2.29 *Measuring height.*

To allow any conclusions to be drawn about physical health from the weight of a person, we obviously need to have an idea of their *height* too. In the example above, you would have formed a different opinion of Paul's physical health if you had been told that he was 1.83 m or 1.60 m. Height should be measured as shown in Fig. 2.29.

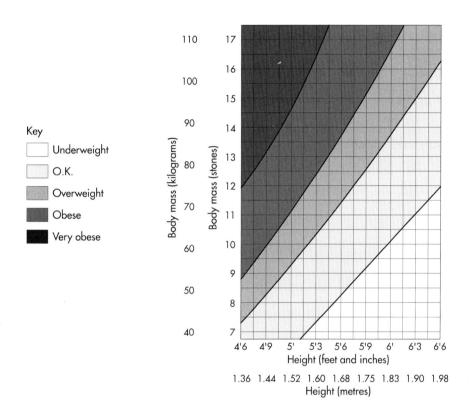

FIGURE 2.30 *Are you a healthy weight?*

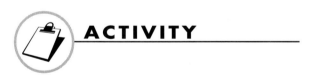

ACTIVITY

Figure 2.30 shows the relationship between weights and heights.

1 Take a straight line across from your height and a line up from your weight. (When you weigh yourself take 2kg off to allow for your clothes.) Check which category you fit into. Does this mean you need to alter your diet/exercise regime? If so, how?

2 Looking at Figure 2.31, what advice would you give to the following people about their diet/exercise based on their weights and heights?

● Palin: 65 kg/1.55 m

● Kate: 47 kg/1.68 m

● Peter: 70 kg/1.75 m

(see end of Chapter for answers.)

Body Mass Index

Body Mass Index is a measure which takes into account both height and weight. It can, therefore, be used to indicate whether a person's weight is healthy for their height.

Body mass index (BMI) is given by the equation:

$$\text{BMI} = \frac{\text{Mass (kg)}}{(\text{Height/m})^2}$$

This means that to calculate your BMI you should:

i) Use your calculator to find the square of your height in metres. (For example, a height of 1.63 m will have a squared value of $1.63 \times 1.63 = 2.83 \text{m}^2$)

ii) Divide your mass in kg by the value calculated in step (i). This gives your BMI.

iii) Compare your calculated BMI with the values given below:

BODY MASS INDEX	INTERPRETATION
Below 20	Underweight
20 – 25	Ideal weight
25.1 – 30	Overweight
Above 30	Obese

Note: Research projects which would involve asking people their weights should be avoided, as some may feel very uncomfortable giving this information.

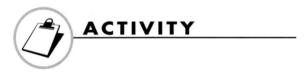 **ACTIVITY**

1 Table 2.9. shows the height and weight of three 18-year old students. For each of them calculate their BMI and say which of them are overweight. (See end of Chapter for Answers.)

	HEIGHT (M)	MASS (KG)
Guy	1.60	74
Heather	1.50	54
Rachel	1.75	77

TABLE 2.9 *Height and mass of three 18 year old students.*

2 Read the article from The Times (27/4/99)/ What would be:

i)   the main advantage and,

ii) the main disadvantage, of using waist measurement to diagnose obesity? (See end of Chapter for answers).

How to tape obesity's measure

People who worry about their weight have made a trip to the bathroom scales the second most urgent task each morning. There is now a simpler regime and a tape measure is all that is needed.

Once the girth of the waist is known doctors should have an immediate idea whether they are dealing with a problem of obesity and, if so, how bad it is.

It has now been shown that a simple waist measurement is all that is needed to assess obesity. Women should have a waist measurement of not more than 32in (80cm) and men 37in (94cm). As long as they keep within these parameters, they don't have to worry too much about having pudding. Doctors will start to get concerned about a female patient if her waist measurement reaches 35in (88cm) or a man has a waistband of 40in (I102cm) or above.

Doctors good at mental arithmetic still like to work out the BMI (the body mass index), which is calculated by dividing the patient's weight in kilograms by his or her height in metres squared. If the BMI is more than 25, the patient has exceeded the recommended calculation and is considered overweight, if more than 30, he or she is technically obese and if the figure is more than 40, grossly obese.

The Times 27/4/99

Peak Flow

Peak flow is a measure of how fast you can blow air out of your lungs. It can be measured with a peak flow meter (Fig. 2.32. When you blow into a peak flow meter it measures the speed of air passing through the meter. This figure is given in cubic decimetres, dm^3, (ie. litres) per minute. Peak flow readings vary according to sex, age, height and even the time of day the measurements taken.

- Peak flow readings are usually higher in men than women.
- The taller a person is, the higher their peak flow is likely to be.
- Peak flow is often higher in the morning than in the evening.

Peak flow measurements are often used to diagnose and monitor the severity of asthma. People with asthma have narrowed airways taking air to the lungs. This may be because the linings of the airways are swollen, or if their is mucus in the airways, or if the tubes are constricted by the muscles surrounding the airways. All of these reduce the amount of air which can flow through the airways. This means that asthma sufferers will have a low peak flow reading, and the more severe their asthma, the lower their reading. Asthma sufferers will have a peak flow reading of 200–400 dm/min. compared with a normal value of 400–60 dm/min. Because peak flow may vary tremendously from time to time, a one-off reading at a surgery may not give a doctor or nurse sufficient information. The asthma sufferer will, therefore, be asked to take their own readings morning and evening over a period of time and plot them on a chart (Fig. 2.33).

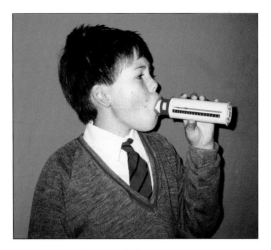

FIGURE 2.31 *Peak flow meter.*

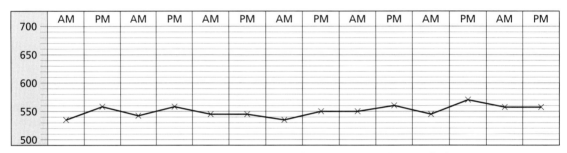

1. Peak flow chart of a person without asthma or a person whose asthma is well controlled

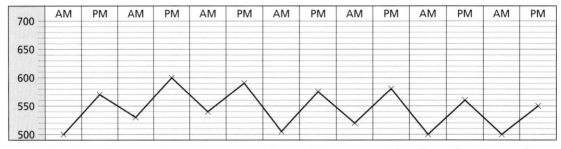

1. Peak flow chart of a person whose asthma is not well controlled   Copyright: Allen and Hamburys Ltd. 1990

FIGURE 2.32 *Peak flow charts.*

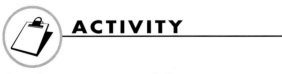 **ACTIVITY**

If you have access to a peak flow meter carry out an investigation into how height affects peak flow.

i) **First write down a *hypothesis* (In other words, a guess at what your results will show).**

ii) **Draw a diagram of the peak flow meter and label it to show how it works. Collect measurements of height and peak flow from at least ten people. (Remember to try to keep other variables constant. For example, take measurements from people who are the same age and the same sex.) Put your results into a table.**

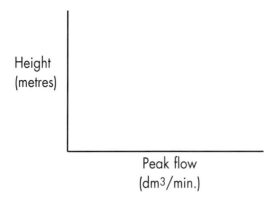

FIGURE 2.33 *Axes for plotting your scattergram.*

iii) Plot a *scattergram* using axes for your graph as shown in Fig. 2.33. (Each person's height and peak flow reading will be plotted as a single point, so you will end up with the same number of points as people measured.)

iv) Are the points arranged randomly or can you fit a 'line of best fit'? If you can, this suggests that there is a *correlation* between height and peak flow.

v) If height and peak flow tend to increase together, we say there is a *positive* correlation. However, if as height increases, peak flow tends to decrease, we say there is a *negative* correlation. If your results show a correlation, is it a positive or negative correlation?

vi) Look back at your hypothesis. Do your results support your hypothesis or not?

....

Resting pulse rate and recovery after exercise

The pumping action of the heart causes a regular pulsation in the blood flow. This can be felt by pressing two finger tips against either the wrist just below the base of the thumb or on the neck a few centimetres below the jaw. It is often most convenient to count for 15 seconds and multiply by four to calculate the number of beats per minute. The pulse rate corresponds to the heart rate which varies according to the person's state of relaxation or physical activity.

Resting pulse rate

The resting pulse rate is the pulse rate taken after a period of relaxation. It should be taken at least three times and an average (mean) calculated. A low resting pulse rate generally indicates a better physical fitness level than a person with a higher resting pulse rate.

- In reasonably fit individuals pulse rate will be between 60 and 60 beats per minute, and on average 72 beats per minute in adults.
- In children and the elderly it will be higher than in young adults.
- Men on average have lower pulse rates than women.
- In top distance athletes it could be as low as 40 beats per minute.

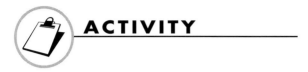

ACTIVITY

1   Take the resting pulse rate of at least three people who regularly take exercise (for example, people who compete regularly in a sport) and three people who take very little exercise. Allow each person at least 5 minutes of relaxation before counting their pulse. Count for 15 seconds and multiply by four to give you pulse rate in Beats per Minute. Don't forget to make three counts of each person's pulse and calculate their mean pulse rate:

$$\text{(Mean pulse rate} = \frac{\text{Pulse rate 1. + Pulse rate 2 + Pulse rate 3)}}{3}$$

2   Plot a bar graph to show the mean pulse rate of each person. Shade the bars to distinguish between the pulse rates of people who exercise and the pulse rates of those who do not.

3   Do your results show lower resting pulse rates in the people who take more exercise? If not, suggest reasons for any unexpected results. For example, it is difficult to measure the amount of exercise people take; there are many factors other than exercise which affect fitness.

Recovery after exercise

Another way of using pulse rate as an indicator of the level of a person's physical fitness is to see how quickly after a period of exercise a person recovers and gets back to their own normal pulse rate.

A **fitness index** can be calculated to measure a person's ability to recover after exercise.

Equipment: Step/bench/ or box 50 cm high; stop watch; metronome or tape with 2 second bleeps.

Procedure: If possible, work in pairs. Step up and down on the step, as shown in Fig. 2.36,at the rate of 30 steps per minute (One step should take two seconds). Ask your partner to check that you are stepping at the correct rate. If you can, keep on stepping for four minutes. If you find this too much, stop, sit down and your partner should write down how many seconds you have managed (out of a total of 240). Rest in a sitting position for sixty seconds. Your partner should then take your pulse for thirty seconds while you remain sitting and then write down the number of beats. Continue resting for a further thirty seconds, and then have your pulse taken again for thirty seconds. Write down the number of beats,. Sit for another thirty seconds and then have your pulse counted for a final thirty seconds. Write down the number of beats **(By now you will have had your pulse taken for thirty seconds one, two, and three minutes after finishing exercise.)**

Calculations:

Time of exercise   = 4 minutes = 240 seconds (or less if you had to stop earlier)

Total number of pulse counts   = Pulse count 1 + Pulse count 2 + Pulse count 3

(For example: 80 + 70 + 60)

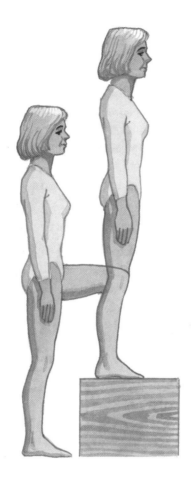

FIGURE 2.34 *The Fitness Index Step Test*

$$\text{Score} = \frac{\text{Time of Exercise in seconds} \times 100}{\text{Total pulse counts} \times 2}$$

For example:
$$\frac{240 \times 100}{(80 + 70 + 60) \times 2}$$

Compare your score with those shown in table 2.10.

FITNESS INDEX SCORE	RATING
90 and over	Excellent
80 – 89	Good
65 – 79	Fair
55 – 69	Poor
54 and below	Very poor

TABLE 2.10 *Fitness Index Scores*

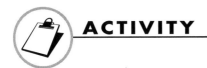

ACTIVITY

i) Take your resting pulse rate twice and record the lowest score. Do five minutes of step exerciser as explained above. After completing the exercise wait for one minute and then take your pulse rate. (Take it for thirty seconds and then multiply by two to give you pulse rate in beats per minute.) Continue taking your pulse rate at intervals of one minute until your pulse rate returns to normal Plot the recovery to the resting rate on a graph. (ie. Plot pulse rate against time on a line graph. In a different colour on the same graph draw a straight line to show your resting pulse rate.)

- How many minutes does it take for your pulse rate to return to the resting rate?
- Find the ratio of your resting pulse rate relative to your pulse rate after exercise. (eg. 70 beats per minute at rest relative to 140 beats after exercise, gives a ratio of 70:140, or 1:2.)

Producing Plans for Promoting Health and Well–Being

For the assessment of this unit you need to produce a plan for promoting health and well–being for a person who is at risk. Below are opportunities to allow you to do this.

● CASE STUDY ● CASE STUDY ● CASE STUDY ● CASE STUDY ● CASE STUDY ● CASE STUDY ●

JOHN – Lifestyle information

John is 52. Three years ago he was made redundant from his job working in a factory. Now he works in a pub five nights a week. He is usually cheerful and enjoys a good social life at work. He is divorced and lives alone. He will sometimes fry himself some food, but generally he snacks at home and relies on pub food, such as pie and chips, in the evening. He smokes about twenty cigarettes a day and usually drinks about five pints of beer a day. He walks a short distance to the bus stop where he catches a bus to work which is about a mile from where he lives, but does very little other exercise.

Measures of health:

The following measurements were recorded for John at a recent physical examination:

Height: 1.75 m
Weight: 102 kg
Peak flow: 510 dm³/min
Resting pulse rate: 88 beats per min

Pulse rate after 4 minutes exercise:

Time (min) after exercise:	Pulse rate (beats per 30 seconds):
1	85
2	76
3	67

Any other observations: John's father died from a heart attack, and his brother suffers from heart trouble.

ANNA – Lifestyle information

Anna is a 25 year old accountant. She has a good income and has recently bought a flat where she lives alone. She finds her work stressful. Because she works such long hours and is exhausted when she gets home, she complains that her social life is non–existent. She is too tired to cook when she gets in, and tends to have a quick glass of wine and snack in front of the TV before falling into bed. At weekends she spends most of her time revising for accountancy exams.

Measures of health:

The following measurements were recorded for Anna at her physical examination:

Height:	1.60 m
Weight:	42 kg
Peak flow:	475 dm³/min
Resting pulse rate:	82 beats per min

Pulse rate after 4 minutes exercise:

Time (min) after exercise:	Pulse rate (beats per 30 seconds):
1	78
2	60
3	48

Any other observations: *Anna complains of usually feeling tense and finding it difficult to relax.*

LIZ – Lifestyle information

Liz is a 17 year old Health and Social Care student. In the week she is at college and spends most evenings either doing course work or working on the check out in a local supermarket. At weekends she relaxes by going out with her friends, either to parties or local night–clubs. Although she does not drink during the week, she often drinks heavily at the weekends and sometimes cannot remember incidents from the night before. She sometimes uses cannabis.

Measures of health:

The following measurements were recorded for Liz at her physical examination:

Height:	1.70 m
Weight:	60 kg
Peak flow:	510 dm³/min
Resting pulse rate:	75 beats per min

● **CASE STUDY** ● **CASE STUDY** ● **CASE STUDY** ● **CASE STUDY** ● **CASE STUDY** ● **CASE STUDY** ● ─

LIZ – Lifestyle information: (continued)

Pulse rate after 4 minutes exercise:

Time (min) after exercise:	Pulse rate (beats per 30 seconds):
1	62
2	48
3	4838

Any other observations: Liz wishes she had time to do more exercise.

Instead of, or as well as, using any of the case studies above, you could prepare a health plan for one of the following:

● **yourself**

● **a person you know** who would be willing to answer questions on their lifestyle and allow you to make simple health measurements. Issues of confidentiality, for example, will you need to change their name?)

● **a named character from a TV 'soap'**

Write an account of the lifestyle and include health measurements as for the case studies. (For the TV character, you will, of course, not be able to make health measurements, but you may be able to make observations about their health.)

To Produce the Health Plan

● Calculate BMI and Fitness Index (page 214).

● Identify any factors which are having a positive effect on physical, social and emotional health.

● Identify risks to physical, social and emotional health, highlighting the ones over which the individual may have control.

● Prioritise long and short term targets for improvement, including timescales.

● Explain the physical, social and emotional effects on the person of achieving the targets.

● Explain in a way appropriate to your chosen person how they can change their behaviour to meet the targets.

● Identify potential difficulties in achieving the plan, and propose realistic ways in which they may be overcome.

● Select health promotional materials, explaining why they were chosen and others were rejected and analysing the ways in which the chosen materials will support the plan.

References and Resources
BOOKS

Aggleton, P. (1990) *'Health'* Publ. Routledge. London ISBN 0-415-00816-6

Blaxter, M. (1990) *'Health and Lifestyles'* Publ. Tavistock/Routledge London.
ISBN 0-415-00147-1

Ewles, L. and Simnett, I (1995) *'Promoting Health – A practical guide. 3rd Edn.'* Publ. Scutari
Press. London. ISBN 1-873853-17-3.

MAFF (1995) *'Manual of nutrition'* The Stationery Office book shops
(Appendix 6 provides a list of the composition of over 200 foods.)

Pike, S. and Forster, D. (1995) *'Health Promotion for All'* Publ Churchill Livingstone London.
ISBN 0-443-05089-9

Secretary of State for Health (1998) *'Our Healthier Nation'* Government Green Paper. London.
The Stationery Office Book shops.

Vellacott, J. and Side, S. (1998) *'Understanding Advanced Human Biology'*
Published by Hodder and Stoughton. ISBN 0340 679115

USEFUL ADDRESSES, PHONE NUMBERS, AND EMAIL ADDRESSES

Action on Smoking and Health (ASH)
This is an American based organisation which has a website – http://ash.org.

Alcohol Concern
This is the UK national agency of alcohol misuse.
Address: Waterbridge House, 32–36 Loman Street, London SE1 OEE
Tel: 020 7928 7377 Fax: 020 7928 4644 Website: www.alcoholconcern.org.uk

Alcoholics Anonymous
You can look for your local branch of the AA in your telephone directory.
Its website is: www.alcoholics-anonymous.org

Central Drugs Prevention Unit
Home Office, Room 354, Horseferry House, Dean Ryle Street, London SW1P 2AW.
Tel. 020 7 217 8631.
(Will provide a wall chart free of charge which illustrates the major drugs of misuse, and drug
taking equip;ment.)

Contraceptive Education Service 020 7636 7866
(For general advice on contraception, or how to find a clinic.)

Drinkline
(National Alcohol Helpline – Gives confidential advice and information about drinking.)
Tel. 0345 32 02 02
All calls charged at local rates. Monday – Friday: 9.30am – 11pm
Saturday and Sunday: 6pm – 11pm

The Food Standards Agency (FSA)
A new public body which gives information to consumers to allow them to make informed choices about the food they eat.

The **Health Development Agency**, Trevelyan House, 30 Great Peter St., London SW1P 2HW. Tel: 020 7413 1985/1987. Enquiries can be e-mailed to the HDA Enquiry Desk on: hda.enquirydesk@hda-online.org.uk. Website: www.hda-online.org.UK

This agency has replaced the **Health Education Authority**. It's aim is to boost the status of public health by advising on good practice and commissioning new research.

The Information Service, The Wellcome Building, 183 Euston Road, London NW1 2BE. Tel: 020 7611 8722. Fax: 020 7611 8726. E-mail: infoserv@wellcome.ac.uk (A medical science information service provided by the Wellcome Trust which consists of a collection of printed, video and computerised information.)

The National Aids Helpline 0800 567 123
(A free, 24 hour confidential service that won't show up on your 'phone bill. Can also give advice on other sexually transmitted diseases.)

National Asthma Campaign
Providence House, Providence Place, London N1 ONT
Telephone: 020 7226 2260
Fax: 020 7704 0740
(Can provide information on Peak Flow measurements.)

National Asthma Campaign Scotland
21 Coates Crescent, Edinburgh EH4 7AF
Telephone: 0131 226 2544
Fax: 0131 226 2401.
Website: http:/www/asthma.org.uk

Asthma Helpline 0345 01 02 03 Open Monday to Friday 9am to 7pm (Calls charged at local rates. Advice by a team of specialist asthma nurses.)

The National Drugs Helpline 0800 77 66 00 – In Welsh on 080037 11 41. (This gives free, 24 hour confidential advice about drugs, including how to talk to children about drugs, counselling, or information on anything to do with drugs. It can give information about local services available in your area.)

Scientific Advisory Committee on Nutrition I(SACN)
This reports to the Food Standards Agency (see above) and the Department of Health.

INTERNET

It is impossible to provide a comprehensive list of websites as the Internet is too large, and is growing and changing too rapidly for this. Some of the useful current sites are listed below, but you will also be able to find many relevant sites yourself.

Health Education Authority (now disbanded) websites:

www.HealthCentral.com
This provides information on:

- Alcohol and substance abuse
- Diet and nutrition
- Sexual health
- Exercise and fitness
- Stress management

It also allows you to create your own health profile by answering a number of questions on your life style. It identifies your greatest health risks and provides helpful links to other health related websites.

www.active.org.uk
Helps people think about how active they are. Plenty of information and suggestions about becoming more active.

www.cyberdiet.com
This site:

- gives the nutrient content of foods
- gives daily nutrient and energy intake recommendations
- allows you to calculate BMI (see page 00)
- sets goals for weight loss
- gives target heart rates during exercise

www.d-code.co.uk
All about D-Code, the HEA's award winning drugs education CD ROM. This site allows you to experience sections online and to order a copy by e-mail.

www.diettalk.com
Gives motivation and encouragement. Reviews of different diets.

www.hawnhs.hea.org.uk
Provides guidance for health authorities, trusts and primary care organisations that want to implement a workplace strategy. Includes advice on: complying with health and safety legislation, improving staff morale, reducing sickness absence, controlling stress, improving recruitment and retention and meeting NHS Executive human resources targets (Working Together).

www.hea.org.uk/locate
Provides free information for professionals on out-of-school drug education and prevention activities for 11–25 year olds in England. Supports local providers, purchasers and planners by putting them in touch with others around the country. The reports available on this site can be used to find out more about drug education and prevention in practice.

www.healthyideas.com/weight
Gives advice on changing long-term eating habits. If weight goal is entered, a meal planner will provide a range of options.

www.lifesafer.co.uk
Offers the support, advice and motivation you may need to stop smoking for life.

www.lovelife.hea.org.uk
The HEA's sexual health website for young people provides up-to-date information on sexual health issues, including how to avoid HIV, other sexually transmitted infections and unwanted pregnancy, and how to use condoms correctly. There is also a quiz and interactive postcards.

www.nutritioncafe.com
This site:

- allows you to analyse the nutrients supplied by different meals;
- gives the nutrient content of different types of food;
- gives a glossary of nutrition terms.

www.thinkfast.co.uk
Website for young people giving fast food facts and a quiz show.

www.trashed.co.uk
A website giving straightforward information about drugs, the risks and what the law says.

www.wad.hea.org.uk
An annual website explaining the Worlds AIDS day.

www.weight.com
Many facts on weight loss, diet and exercise, plus you can ask your own questions.

www.wrecked.co.uk
An interactive website for young people exploring alcohol issues.

www.ag.uiuc.edu/food-lab-nat/
The Nutrition Analysis Tool (NAT) is a web-based programme, which allows you to calculate the nutrient content of your diet.

ww.agricola.umn.edu/nutritiontools/kcalculator.cfm
This will calculate your energy requirements based on BMI and energy expenditure.

SOFTWARE

There are computer programmes which can be used to analyse diet. For example, 'Analyse your diet' can be obtained from: AVP Computing, School Hill Centre, Chepstow, Gwent NP6 5PH Tel. (01291) 625439 Fax (01291) 279671

LEAFLETS

A number of useful leaflets on actors either contributing to a healthy lifestyle, or putting health at risk can generally be found in the following:

- supermarkets
- chemists
- health centres and Doctor's surgeries
- libraries

(NB. Check who has published the leaflet as they may be biased. For example, organisations such as food manufacturers may be trying to present their products in a good light!)

Health Education Authority with the Department of Health and MAFF (1996).
'The balance of good health' ISBN 0 7521 0634 1
(Copies of this leaflet may be obtained from local Health Promotion Units and Departments.)

LOCAL ORGANISATIONS

There will be a number of organisations found in your particular area which may be able to provide you with published information, or even send a speaker to your school or college or give you the opportunity for visits or work experience. Look in telephone directories or ask at your local library for details. The suggestions below may give you some ideas:

- local health promotion units
- local Drugs Advisory Service
- local drug action teams
- specialists from local hospitals or health centres, such as health visitors or dieticians, may be able to provide specialist input on some topics.

Glossary

Anorexia Nervosa – An eating disorder, characterised by severe weight loss.

Body Mass Index (BMI) – A simple assessment of body mass.

$$BMI = \frac{body\ mass/kg}{(height/m)^2}$$

Chronic Condition – A disease of long duration involving very changes. It often starts very gradually.

Disease – A specific condition of ill health. Identified as an actual change on the surface, or inside, some part of the body.

Drug – Any chemical substance which changes the function of one or more body organs or alters the process of the disease.

Emotional Health – Concerned with being able to express feelings such as fear, joy, grief, frustration and anger. It also includes the ability to cope with anxiety, stress, and depression,

Health – See pages 163–169

Health Education – Any activity which promotes health-related learning.

Health Promotion – The process of enabling people to increase their control over, and to improve, their health.

Hygiene – This is concerned with preventing disease causing organisms entering the body.

Illness – The subjective state of feeling unwell. (i.e. How people feel). (Compare with 'Disease' and 'Sickness'.)

Intellectual Health – This is concerned with the ability to think clearly and rationally. It is closely linked to emotional and social health.

Obesity – The excessive deposit of fat under the skin.

Pathogen – Disease causing organism, for example, bacteria or viruses.

Peak Flow – The maximum speed at which air can be forced out of the lungs.

Physical Health – This is concerned with the physical functioning of the body. It is the easiest aspect of health to measure.

Sickness – Reported illness. Involves being treated by a professional and becoming a medical statistic.

Social Class – A way of differentiating between groups and individuals within society, usually using professional and employment status.

Social Health – This is concerned with the ability to relate to others and to form relationships.

Answers

Diet

How much energy is needed?
Energy requirements depend on:

- age (size)
- sex
- activity levels

Foods most commonly causing allergies:

- food additives
- shellfish
- nuts (particularly peanuts)

What should be done:
Seek specialist advice from a dietician.

Reasons for the elderly neglecting their diet:

- low income
- poor mobility
- poor appetite
- apathy and depression (eg. if living alone)
- reluctance to change habits

(You may think of other equally valid answers.)

Social Class
Activity 2. i)

- High fat foods are often cheaper than more 'healthy' foods.
- High fat foods may be more readily available than, for example, fresh fruit and vegetables.
- People may not have information about healthy diets.
- Many forms of exercise are expensive and chid care may not be available.
- Important issues such as housing and employment may take priority over 'healthy' eating and exercise.

ii) There are many other reasons for ill-health which will have more impact on people from lower social classes, for example, poverty, unemployment, and poor housing.

Employment
Activity 2.

Employment can benefit a person in a number of ways, other than providing an income. For example, some types of employment which involve physical activity may contribute to fitness;a person may feel intellectually stimulated by their employment; it is likely that employment will provide opportunities for socialising and friendship.

Housing
Activity 1.

HEALTH PROBLEM	CAUSE(S)
Asthma	Damp
Bad back	Carrying pushchair/child upstairs
Diarrhoea	Inadequate food storage; Poor washing facilities (overcrowded and lack of hot water after 10 pm); Possibly lack of hygiene in mobile food van.
Depression	Overcrowding causing stress: Lack of social contact.

Income
Advantage of minimum wage:
Prevent exploitation of workers.
Disadvantages of minimum wage:
May mean employers can afford to employ fewer workers; may be difficult to enforce.

Education
Activity 2
Ways in which pregnancy could cause poor education could include: time missed from school during, and immediately after the pregnancy,; cost of childcare means mother's education cut short; combining studying and childcare is exhausting.

Illegal drug use
Activity 2
What to do if you find someone very drowsy or unconscious because of drug taking:

1 Don't panic.
2 Make sure they've got plenty of fresh air.
3 Try not to leave them alone in case they vomit and choke.
4 Dial 999 and ask for an ambulance.
5 Collect up anything that seems to have been used in the drug taking and give them to a member of the ambulance crew.

Sexual behaviour quiz

1 d)
2 b)
3 g)

Unsafe practices in the workplace

- books balanced precariously
- poor light
- no fire extinguisher
- blocked fire exit
- lifting heavy box
- boiling kettle with trailing flex
- someone standing on a swivel chair
- 1st aid box with contents spilling out
- tipping filing cabinet

Measuring
Activity 1.
Palin: Overweight. Action: Increase exercise / Cut back on fats in diet
Kate: Underweight. Action: A higher energy diet is required.
Peter: O.K.

BMI
Activity 1.
Guy	29 (overweight)
Heather	24 (ideal weight)
Rachel	25 (ideal weight)

Activity 2.
Main advantage: Quick and easy. No calculations.
Main disadvantage: Takes no account of taller people having larger waists.

C H A P T E R 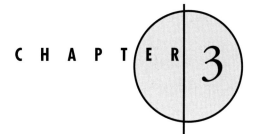 3

Understanding personal development

Introduction

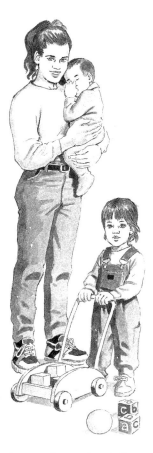

Carers who work with people need to know about the different ways that people grow and develop and the different factors, including social, environmental and biological factors, which can contribute to growth and development.

After working through this chapter you should:

➡ understand the physical, social, intellectual and emotional growth that takes place throughout life;

➡ know how social and economic factors can affect development;

➡ have learnt about factors which affect self–concept (the way we see ourselves);

➡ know examples of life–changes and be able to describe the positive or negative effects of these changes;

➡ know the types of support available to help a person cope with change;

➡ know how to identify the physical, intellectual, emotional and social needs of a person in order to provide appropriate support.

Human growth and development

● **Growth** is an increase in size and complexity.

● **Development** is the process of gaining new skills.

Milestones, or **norms**, show what most children can do at a particular age. However, it is important to remember that although using norms helps us to understand patterns of development, each child will, of course, develop in their own unique way and there will be wide variation between individuals. Keep this in mind when using the development tables below.

Throughout a person's life, growth and development should be considered under the following headings:

● *P*hysical

● *I*ntellectual

● *E*motional

● *S*ocial

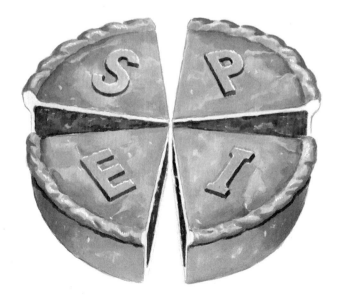

FIGURE 3.1 *'PIES' – Personal, Intellectual, Emotional and Social development.*

Remember! The word '*pies*' should help you learn these headings. See Figure 3.1 and p. 31 of the Study Skills Guide. Each type of development is described below. Growth and development takes place during each of the five main life stages.

LIFE STAGE	APPROXIMATE AGE RANGE
Infancy	0–1 years
Childhood	2–10 years
Puberty and Adolescence	11–late teens
Adulthood	20–65
Old Age	65 and beyond

TABLE 3.1 *The five main life stages*

Growth

GROWTH IN INFANCY

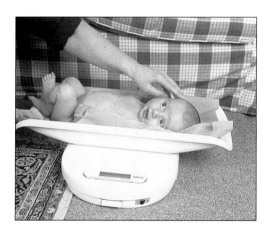 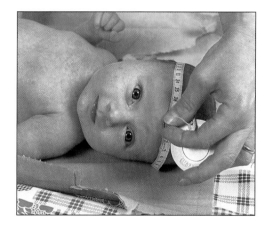

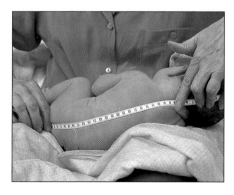

FIGURE 3.2 *Photographs of weighing a baby, measuring the length of a baby and measuring the head circumference of a baby.*

There are various ways of measuring the growth of a baby, (see Figure 3.2). The three measurements most commonly made are:

- weight
- length
- head circumference

A new–born baby, on average:

- weighs 3.5 kg
- has a length of about?
- has a head circumference of about 35 cm

Boys are, on average, about 100g heavier than girls, and slightly longer.

The body parts of a baby do not all grow at the same rate. For example, in the first year:

- the **legs** and **arms** grow at a **faster** rate than the rest of the body;

- the **head** grows at a **slower** rate than the rest of the body.

Figure 3.3 shows how the differences in growth rates of the various parts of the body lead to changes in the proportions of the body.

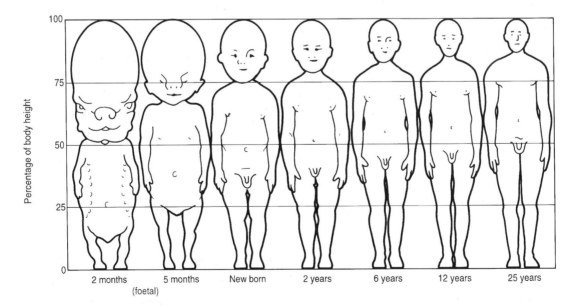

FIGURE 3.3 *The proportions of the body change throughout life.*

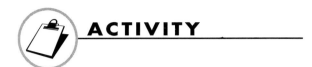

ACTIVITY

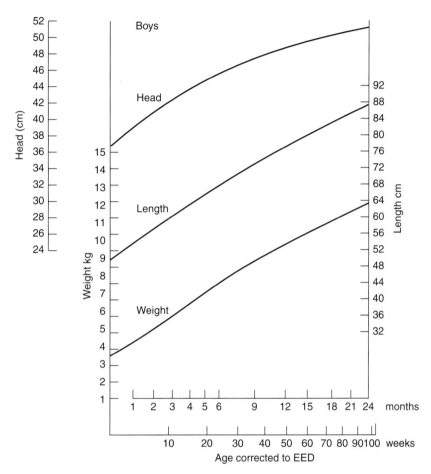

FIGURE 3.4 *Average weights, lengths and head circumference of boy babies.*

1 Figure 3.4 shows the average weights, lengths and head circumferences of boy babies.
   (i)   Look at this figure and work out how long it takes for an average baby to double its birth weight. (Give your answer to the nearest month). (See end of Chapter for Answers.)
   (ii) Many health authorities issue parents with a 'Personal Health Record' book to record measurements of their babies. If possible, have a look at one of these books.
2 You may be able to arrange to observe a health visitor weighing babies at a local clinic. This activity would obviously not be suitable for a whole class, but may be possible for one or two students at a time.

GROWTH IN CHILDHOOD

By the time a child is three years old, their weight is generally about four times their birth weight (see Figure 3.4). Figure 3.5 shows the growth rate between the ages of 2 and 9 years old. During this time growth takes place at a fairly constant rate, and at a slower rate than the growth between 0–1 years.

The skull and brain have usually reached adult size by the time the child is about 5, but after this the child's appearance changes as the upper and lower jaws grow rapidly, and the first set of teeth are replaced by the permanent teeth.

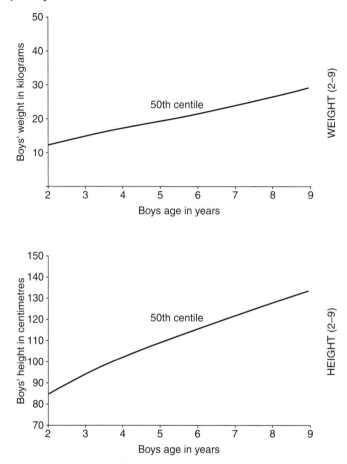

FIGURE 3.5 *a) Average weights of boys (2–9 years).*
b) Average heights of girls (2–9 years).

GROWTH IN PUBERTY AND ADOLESCENCE

In adolescence there is a sudden increase in growth rate and maturity. This produces an adult who would be able to produce and care for young.

Adolescence starts with puberty, which is the time during which **secondary sexual characteristics** develop (see Figure 3.6.) Puberty usually starts at about 10 in girls, and 12 in boys. By the late teens, the changes are usually complete.

The increase in growth rate in adolescence is known as the **second growth spurt**. This is different in males and females.

- In girls the growth spurt usually occurs between about 11 and 12 years old, but in boys it is usually between 13 and 15 years old.
- In boys the growth spurt lasts longer than in girls, which means that men are generally larger than women.

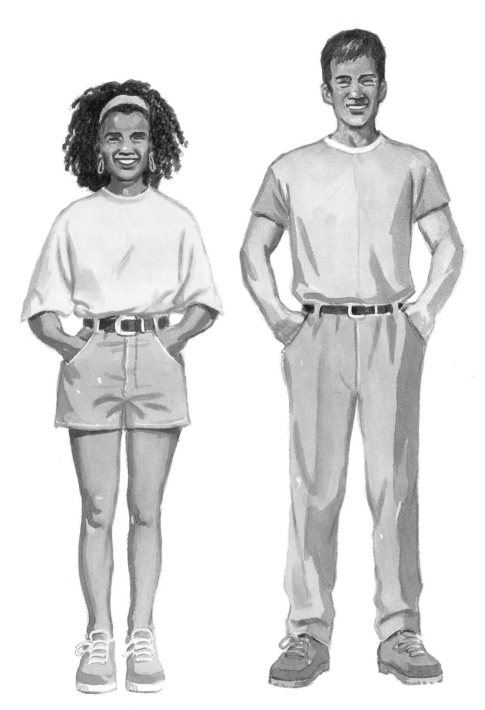

FIGURE 3.6 *Secondary sexual characteristics.*

GROWTH IN ADULTHOOD

By the end of adolescence the body is physically and sexually mature. Although growth no longer takes place, physical changes to the body continue as the body ages.

The **menopause** occurs in women, usually at between 45 and 55 years of age. After this, women do not produce eggs which means they can no longer become pregnant. Men, however, can continue to produce sperm and thus father children into old age.

GROWTH IN OLD AGE

Figure 3.7 shows how the main body systems deteriorate with age. Despite these changes, it is important that elders are encouraged to approach the ageing process with a positive attitude. Improved health care (among other factors) has increased life expectancy and the qualify of life in old age. In addition, their wealth of experience allows elderly people to make valuable contributions (see Figure 3.8.)

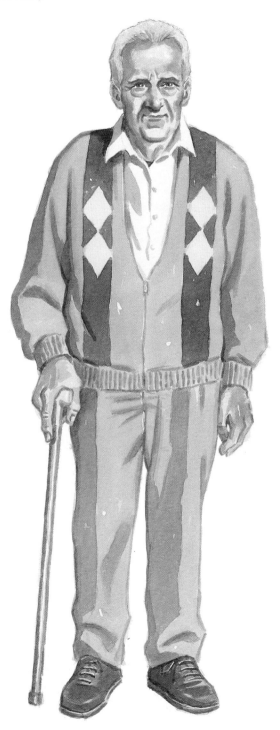

FIGURE 3.7 *The ageing process.*

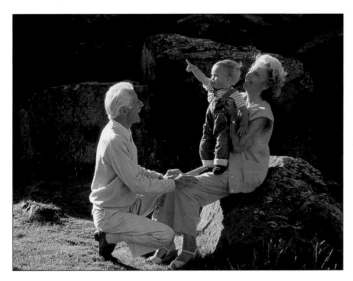

FIGURE 3.8 *Elderly people can use their wealth of experience to make valuable contributions.*

Physical development

Figure 3.9 shows that the physical skills which develop throughout life can be divided into two main areas.

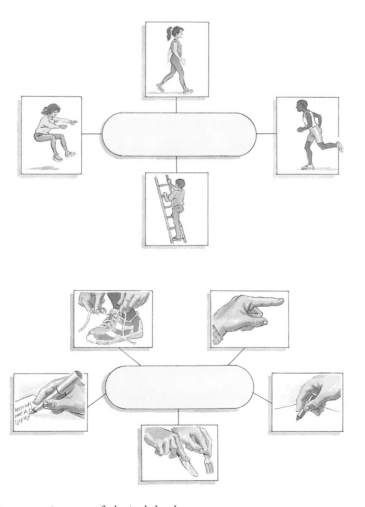

FIGURE 3.9 *The two main areas of physical development.*

PHYSICAL DEVELOPMENT IN INFANCY

Table 3.2 shows the development of both gross motor skills and fine manipulative skills in infancy.

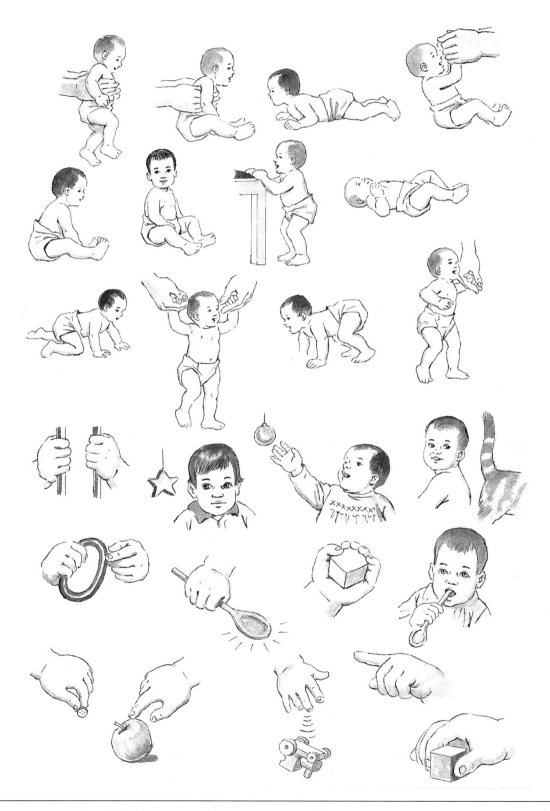

TABLE 3.2 *Physical development in infancy.*

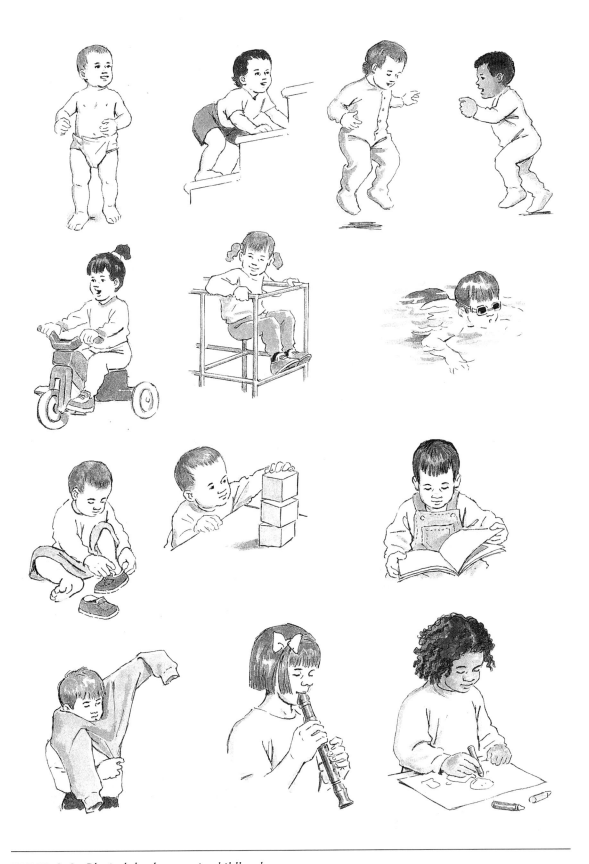

TABLE 3.3 *Physical development in childhood.*

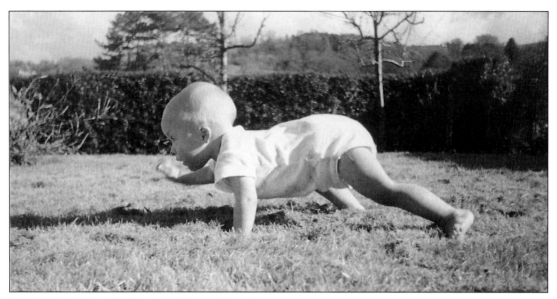

FIGURE 3.10 *"Walking" on feet and hands.*

Table 3.3 shows the development of both gross motor skills and fine manipulative skills in childhood.

PHYSICAL DEVELOPMENT IN PUBERTY AND ADOLESCENCE, ADULTHOOD AND OLD AGE

By the time the nervous system is fully developed, all the main developmental milestones will have been reached. However, even in later life, people may learn new gross motor skills and fine manipulative skills (see Figure 3.11).

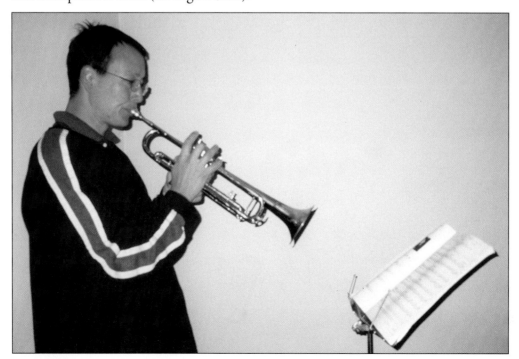

FIGURE 3.11 *New physical skills may still be learnt in adulthood.*

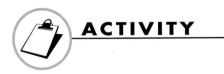

ACTIVITY

1 Read the list below of examples of skills which may be acquired in adulthood. Which are gross motor skills and which are fine manipulative skills?

- Rollerblading
- Embroidery
- Skiing
- Playing the flute (See end of Chapter for Answers.)

2 Can you think of any physical skills you have learned since childhood?

....

Intellectual development

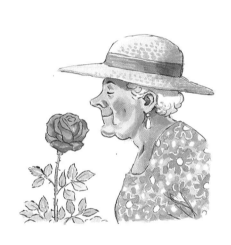

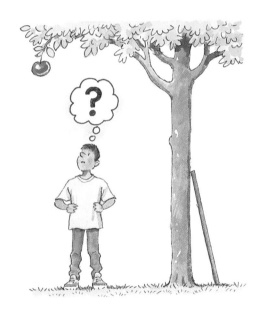

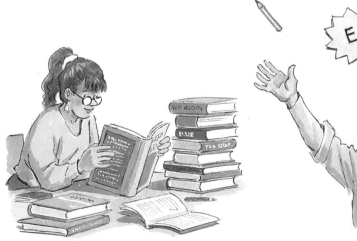

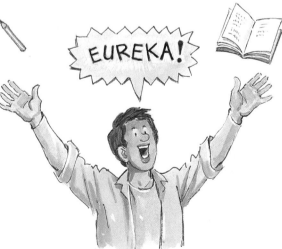

FIGURE 3.12 *Aspects of intellectual development.*

Intellectual development refers to the development of the parts of the brain concerned with:

- perception (absorbing information about the environment through the senses of sight, hearing, touch, smell and taste).
- acquiring knowledge
- reasoning
- understanding

Every brain cell a person has is present at their birth. During childhood the brain grows very quickly. By the age of 1 year, the baby's brain is already three–quarters of its adult size and rapid development continues until middle childhood.

INTELLECTUAL DEVELOPMENT IN INFANCY

Table 3.4 shows some of the stages of intellectual development in infancy.

AGE	DEVELOPMENT
0–4 weeks	Babies receive information about the world through their senses. *Touch* Their faces, abdomens, hands and soles of feet are particularly sensitive. *Hearing* New born babies turn towards a sound. By 2 weeks old they will stop crying and listen to a human voice. *Taste* Like sweet tastes. *Smell* Turn to the smell of the breast. *Sight* Can focus on objects about 200m away, but probably don't see colour. They will initiate facial expressions (Figure 3.13).
4–16 weeks	Recognise different speech sounds. By 3 months they can imitate low or high pitched sounds.
4–5 months	Can reach objects, showing that they can judge distances. Know the difference between two- and three-dimensional objects.
5–6 months	Recognise familiar objects, e.g. feeding bottle. Can coordinate movements such as reaching or grasping. Develop favour tastes in food.
6–9 months	Understands signs (e.g. bib means food is coming) Understands that objects are permanent (e.g.. when a toy is covered with cloth it still exists.)
9 months–1 year	Memory develops. Can anticipate the future, so can understand daily routines. Can imitate events after they have finished. (e.g. initiate a temper tantrum they saw a friend have the day before.)

TABLE 3.4 *Intellectual development Infancy (0–1 year) (Adapted from: "Child Care and Education"*
Bruce & Meggitt. Publ. Hodder & Stoughton 1996).

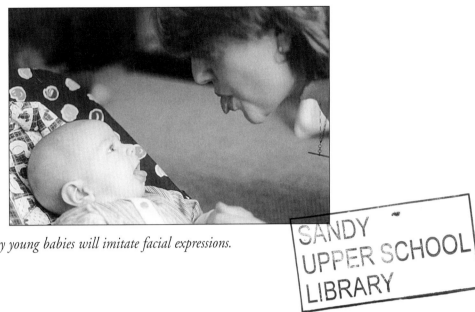

FIGURE 3.13 *Very young babies will imitate facial expressions.*

INTELLECTUAL DEVELOPMENT IN CHILDHOOD

Table 3.5 shows some of the stages of intellectual development in childhood.

AGE	DEVELOPMENT
1–4 years	Talking develops. Pretend play develops (Figure 3.14). Can take part in simple games. Learn to draw and make models. May start to enjoy music. Find it difficult to see things from another's point of view, but this will start to develop.
4–7 years	Language well established. Reading and writing develop (Figure 3.15). Concepts of measurement develop (e.g. length, time, weight). An understanding of number develops. Can help younger children play. Start to develop an understanding of 'right' and 'wrong'.
9 years onwards	Develops an understanding of abstract concepts such as justice, good versus evil.

TABLE 3.5 *Intellectual development: Childhood (1–10 years) (Adapted from: "Child Care and Education:" Bruce & Meggitt. Publ. Hodder & Stoughton 1996).*

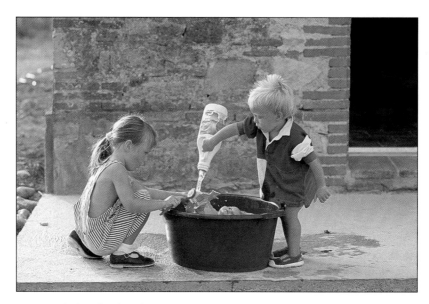

FIGURE 3.14 *Pretend play develops between 0–4 years.*

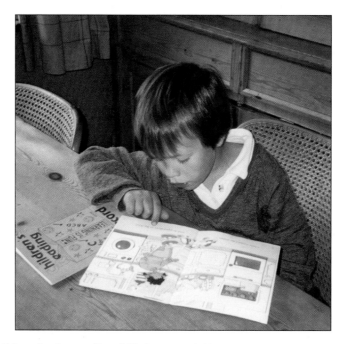

FIGURE 3.15 *Children develop reading skills between 4–7 years.*

INTELLECTUAL DEVELOPMENT FROM PUBERTY AND ADOLESCENCE INTO ADULTHOOD

The way in which adolescents and adults think may differ in a number of ways from the ways children think; For example:

● **thinking about possibilities**: young children rely heavily on their senses to apply reasoning, whereas adolescents are more likely to think about alternative possibilities that are not directly observable.

- **thinking ahead**: adolescence is the time when young people start to plan ahead. Younger children may look forward to a holiday, for example, but are not able to focus on the preparation required.
- **thinking about thought**: adolescents can think about their own thought processes in an increasingly complex way. They are also able to think about other peoples' points of view.
- **thinking beyond conventional limits**: issues such as morality, religion and politics can be discussed with greater complexity by adolescents.

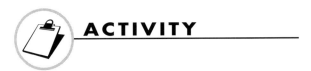

ACTIVITY

Read through the examples above of how an adolescent's or adult's thinking might differ from a child's thinking. For each stage, can you think of examples of occasions on which you have demonstrated this type of thinking?

. . . .

INTELLECTUAL DEVELOPMENT IN OLD AGE

In old age there may be changes in memory, but only in certain aspects. Long established skills, such as money management, playing a musical instrument or gardening, remain unaffected by old age. The memory for names and everyday activities, however, may be affected. Sometimes an older person may find it difficult to distinguish between a real and an imagined event. For example some elderly people may believe they have turned the gas off, when in reality they have only thought about turning it off.

The ability to recall events from the distant past improves slightly into middle age, and by the age of 60 shows only a slight decline.

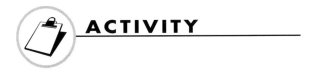

ACTIVITY

Case study

Christine goes to visit her elderly mother who lives very close to her. As she arrives, she finds her mother returning from a visit to the shops. They go into her mother's house together to find that the gas cooker has been left on. A saucepan and its contents have been ruined but there is no lasting damage.

1 How should Christine react?

2 Can you think of strategies to help elderly people remember important actions and events?

. . . .

Emotional and social development

Emotional development involves the development of self–image and identity (see section on self–concept and self–esteem, on p 270) and the ways in which an individual makes sense of emotions in themselves and of feelings towards others.

Social development involves the growth of the individual's relationship with others and the development of social skills. It is impossible to isolate emotional and social development from one another, or from intellectual and physical development.

EMOTIONAL AND SOCIAL DEVELOPMENT IN INFANCY

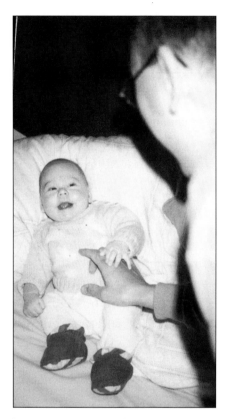

FIGURE 3.16 *Babies will smile at a carer at around 5–6 weeks.*

Table 3.6 shows some of the states in emotional and social development in infancy.

Birth – 4 weeks	Enjoyment of feeding and cuddling. The baby shows pleasure, e.g. at bathtime, with whole body movements.
4–8 weeks	Responds by smiling at an adult (Fig 3.16). Recognises face of preferred adult. Turns towards someone speaking.
8–12 weeks	Longer periods of being awake. Fixes eyes on carer's face when feeding.
4–5 months	Sleep patterns have developed. Knows she has only one mother, and shows distress if several images of the mother are shown at one time.

| 6–9 months | More wary of strangers.
Offers toys to others.
Shows distress when main carer leaves.
Become more aware of other's feelings. e.g. will cry if brother cries; will laugh if others laugh. |
| 9–12 months | Likes to be near familiar adult.
Will play alone for long periods.
Shows definite lies and dislikes, e.g. at mealtime or bedtime.
Imitates other people, e.g. clapping or waving. |

TABLE 3.6 *Emotional and social development: Infancy (0–1 years).*

EMOTIONAL AND SOCIAL DEVELOPMENT IN CHILDHOOD

Table 3.7 shows some of the stages of emotional and social development in childhood.

1–2 years	Starts to learn what hurts and upsets their family, and what brings pleased responses. A longer memory develops. Expresses needs in words and gestures.
2–3 years	Develops ability to say how she is feeling. Pretend play helps a child develop a sense of what other people are feeling.
3–4 years	Becomes aware of being male or female. Makes friends. (Figure 3.17). Learns to negotiate with others.
4–8 years	Can hide feelings. Can think about the feelings of others. Can take responsibility (e.g. will help younger children).

TABLE 3.7 *Emotional and social development: Childhood.*

EMOTIONAL AND SOCIAL DEVELOPMENT IN ADOLESCENCE AND PUBERTY

Adolescence is a period when most young people are working towards their own independence. They want to be able, increasingly, to make their own decisions, test the limits of authority and express their own individuality. It is also a time when peer pressure is at its highest. During the early part of adolescence, young people are likely to be more self–conscious and more self–critical than before.

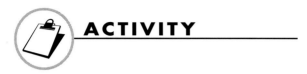

ACTIVITY

Discussion point:

It is said that attractiveness and peer acceptance are seen as more important in the development of self–esteem during adolescence than other factors, such as being good at sports or good at academic subjects. Do you agree with this?

EMOTIONAL AND SOCIAL DEVELOPMENT IN ADULTHOOD

Adulthood has been described as a state of 'maturity'. A mature individual is considered to have the following attributes:

● stable emotional behaviour

● an accurate self–concept (see p 270)

● satisfying relationships

● a realistic estimation of future goals

These attributes will help when it comes to dealing with the inevitable life–changes which will be faced in adulthood (see p 273).

EMOTIONAL AND SOCIAL DEVELOPMENT IN OLD AGE

Three different theories of ageing help to explain some of the emotional and social changes in this period of life:

1 **Erikson's psycho–social theory** suggests that there are two conflicting points of view about old age. These are illustrated in Figure 3.17. Successful ageing depends on the individual adopting the more positive view of ageing.

2 The **social disengagement theory** (Fig. 3.18) suggests that the following social changes take place in old age:

society withdraws from the individual. For example:

➡ there is compulsory retirement, usually at the age of 65;

➡ children grow up, leave home and have families of their own;

➡ friends, or maybe the spouse, die

the individual withdraws from society. For example:

➡ there is a reduction in social contacts and activity;

➡ life becomes more solitary.

It is suggested that the decrease in social and emotional responsibilities in the later years leads to contentment and so these changes are beneficial. Others, however, believe that these changes are harmful and are caused by the negative attitudes in society towards elderly people.

3 The **activity theory** (Fig. 3.19) proposes that successful ageing involves staying active and participating in as many social activities as possible.

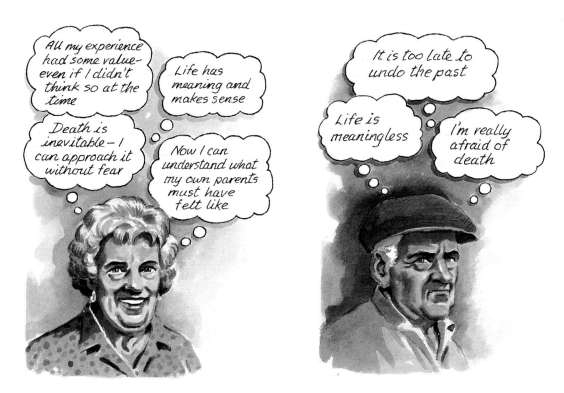

FIGURE 3.17 *Erikson's psychosocial theory – two conflicting points of view about old age.*

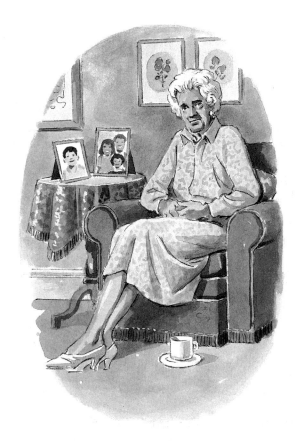

FIGURE 3.18 *Social disengagement theory.*

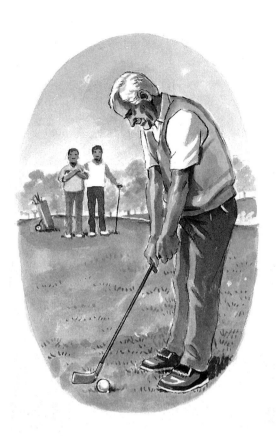

FIGURE 3.19 *Activity theory.*

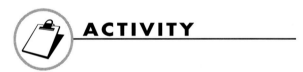

ACTIVITY

Look at Figures 3.18 and 3.19 which illustrate the social disengagement theory and activity theory respectively. From your experience of elderly people, which theory do you think is most accurate?

....

Social and economic factors in personal development

WHAT ARE SOCIAL AND ECONOMIC FACTORS?

The ways in which people grow and develop are not only influenced by biological and physical factors but are affected, within society, by the kind of 'training' for social life people receive (**socialisation**), by their relationships with others and by the access they have to the resources needed for survival.

Social factors which affect personal development therefore describe the patterns in and expectations of social behaviour which may affect, for instance, people's health, their employment prospects, their level of education and their self–esteem. The groups people are part of (families, friends, ethnic, religious or cultural groups, sex and age categories such as young boys or adult women, community, work or school based groups) will have a significant impact upon their lives.

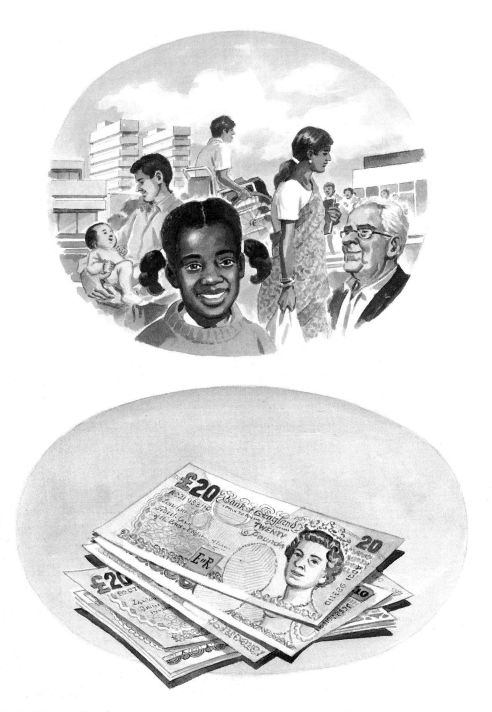

FIGURE 3.20 *Social and economic factors which can influence personal development.*

Economic factors also affect personal development because people need resources (money, income, wealth) to pay for things which are essential, such as food, clothing and housing. People may also want further resources for items which they desire but which are not essential, such as designer–label clothing, meals in restaurants or expensive holidays. The ways in which people are able to obtain and use money will have a significant effect on their health, welfare and self–esteem.

Figure 3.20 illustrates some of the social and economic factors which can influence personal development.

● *CASE STUDY* ● *CASE STUDY* ● *CASE STUDY* ● *CASE STUDY* ● *CASE STUDY* ● *CASE STUDY* ●

Andy

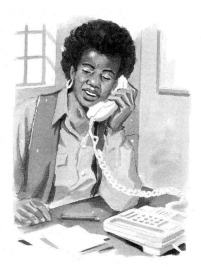
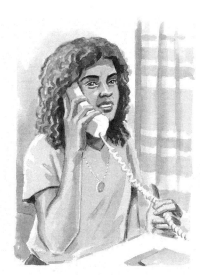

Pat phones her friend Karen. She is in tears. Pat's cousin, Andy, is in hospital, recovering from an attempt to commit suicide. Pat was quite close to Andy but had not realised he was so unhappy. Andy is twenty years old with one younger brother. He lives with his mother who is divorced from his father. He is in the second year of an engineering course at a local college of further education.

Karen wonders whether Andy had any close friends. Was anything happening to him at college or at the shop where he had a part-time job? Was he feeling under pressure at work? Was he taking drugs? Had there been a crisis in his family or social life? Karen discussed these and many more questions with Pat, who needed someone to talk it all over with.

A few days later Pat phoned again and said that she had been talking to Andy and his family. A picture of why he had tried to commit suicide was beginning to develop.

His parent's divorce, six months ago, and the bitter quarrels leading up to it, had depressed and worried Andy. His father was no longer contributing financially to his ex-family and Andy was working part-time for fifteen hours a week or more to help pay for his upkeep and support the family.

Andy's girlfriend, Jessica, had recently finished their relationship, saying that he was always working and was too involved with his family to have an enjoyable social life with her.

Andy's younger brother, Peter, age ten, had severe asthma. Their council house was damp and badly ventilated, which made the illness worse. The family could not afford to move. Andy recently spent the whole weekend in hospital with Peter after he'd had a severe asthma attack.

● CASE STUDY ● CASE STUDY ● CASE STUDY ● CASE STUDY ● CASE STUDY ● CASE STUDY ●

Andy (continued)

The amount of time spent on his part–time job did not give Andy enough time to do this college work. He was often too tired to concentrate in classes. His practical work was badly affected and his grades weren't good. He'd also had to take time off from college for the coughs, sore throats and colds he often suffered from.

FIGURE 3.21 *Case–study: Andy*

ACTIVITY

What social and economic factors might have played a part in Andy's suicide attempt? Use the table below to tick the factors which you think might have applied. Explain how each factor you have ticked might have played a part in his attempted suicide.

SOCIAL AND ECONOMIC FACTORS	TICK	HOW MIGHT THIS FACTOR HAVE PLAYED A PART IN ANDY'S SUICIDE ATTEMPT?
Family		
Friends		
Ethnicity		
Culture		
Gender		
Social class		
Social isolation		
Discrimination		
Stereotyping		
Housing and environment		
Access to services (such as education)		
Income		
Availability of money for essentials		
Availability of money for non-essentials		

TABLE 3.8 *Social and economic factors.*

Further questions to consider

1 Do we always have **control** over the social and economic factors which influence our health and personal development? Which social and economic factors do you think Andy had **most** or **least** control over in the few months leading up to his attempted suicide?

2 Can you think of ways in which Andy could better manage the social and economic influences on his life? Would he need outside help or support? If so, what kinds of support would be available to him? How could his family and friends help him? What changes might he need to consider making in his life?

3 How many 'Andys' are there in the UK today? Carry out research into the extent and nature of attempted and completed suicides among younger people in the U.K. Is attempted suicide/suicide on the increase or decrease? Among which groups of the population is it most common? How might the trends and patterns in suicides be explained?

Game: In the Hot Seat — Wants or Needs?

Step One

Look at the four lists below. You will see that each list contains seven suggestions for the **economic resources** we may **want** or **need** to live healthily and happily in this society.

Step Two

Make one photocopy of page 259 for each small group playing "In the Hot Seat" and cut out the suggestion boxes. Each group should then, after discussion, place each suggestion in one of two piles labelled as follows:

1 Economic resources we **need** to live healthily and happily.

2 Economic resources we may **want** to live healthily and happily.

No suggestion should be placed in any category unless all group members agree. Where there is a difference of opinion, those in the minority in the group should remain, 'in the hot seat' until agreement is reached. Their views should be challenged and questioned by the others and they should have to justify them and attempt to persuade the rest of the group that their choice is the right one. If absolutely no agreement can be reached, the reasons should be recorded by the group and that suggestion omitted from the final piles.

Step Three

A plenary session can follow, where each group tells the others which suggestions they have placed in their lists and differences can be noted and discussed. The whole class can try to decide upon where any omitted suggestions from each group ought to go.

1 Enough income to buy (and replace when worn out/outgrown) a set of basic clothing from second-hand/charity shops or similar, e.g. jumble sales: Approx. **£200.00** per person per year.

1 Enough income to make (sew, knit etc.) most of your own clothes and to buy the rest. Approx. **£300.00** per person per year.

1 Enough income to buy (and replace when worn out/outgrown) a set of new basic clothing from high street stores or equivalent, e.g. mail order. Approx. **£600.00** per person per year.

1 Enough income to buy (and replace when worn out/outgrown) a set of clothing from designer shops/with designer labels. Approx. **£1200.00** per person per year.

---

2 Enough income to afford a weekly food/household goods bill of **£20.00–30.00** per person.

2 Enough income to afford a weekly food/household goods bill of **£30.00–40.00** per person.

2 Enough income to afford a weekly food/household goods bill of **£40.00–50.00** per person.

2 Enough income to afford to spend as much as you like on food and household goods plus restaurant and take-away bills.

---

3 Enough income to afford to buy, after all other essentials have been paid for, up to 4 second-class postage stamps a week. Approx. **£1.00–2.00** per person.

3 Enough income to afford to buy, after all other essentials have been paid for, birthday/Christmas/other religious festival presents for close family. Approx. **£80.00** per person per year

3 Enough income to afford to buy, after all other essentials have been paid for, up to ten units of alcohol a week and/or twenty cigarettes a day. Approx. **£35.00–50.00** per person per week.

3 Enough income to afford to buy personal private health insurance. Between **£500.00–1000.00** per person per year.

---

4 Enough income to buy, insure and maintain a second-hand pedal bicycle with safety helmet and puncture kit. Approx. **£150.00** per person in the year the bicycle is bought.

4 Enough annual income to afford to pay off a monthly loan on, tax, insure, service and buy petrol for a small second-hand car. Approx. **£1800.00** per person in the year the car is bought.

4 Enough annual income to afford to pay off a monthly loan on, tax, insure, service and buy petrol for a small new car. approx. **£4000.00** per person in the year the car is bought.

4 Enough income to afford to buy outright, tax, insure, service and run a new car. Anything above **£12,000.00** in the year the car is bought.

---

5 Enough income to rent a room in a hostel or night shelter

5 Enough income to rent a flat/house from a council, a housing association, private land lord or a co-operative.

5 Enough income to borrow money from a building society, bank or other lender (this is called a mortgage) to buy a house or flat. You will usually be allowed to borrow two and a half to three times your annual gross income, i.e. before tax.

5 Enough income to buy your housing outright.

6 Enough income to afford a weekly T.V. rental payment and annual T.V. licence bill. Approx. **£200.00** a year per person.

6 Enough income to afford to buy a new T.V. and video and pay the annual T.V. licence fee. Approx. **£300.00–400.00** per person in the year the T.V./video were bought.

6 Enough income to buy a home computer and software and pay for fax, e-mail and Internet services plus subscriptions to satellite, cable and digital T.V. Approx. **£1500.00–2000.00** in the year the computer was bought.

6 Enough income to afford to buy outright any combination of T.V., video, computer, fax, games console, software, printers etc. the individual or family desires. Approx. **£5000.00+** in the year the items are bought.

7 Employment pay and/or social security benefit/pension which gives an income (after tax) of **£80.00** plus housing benefit per person per week.

7 Employment pay and/or social security benefit/pension which gives an income (after tax) of **£130.00–250.00** a week.

7 Employment pay and/or social security benefit/pension which gives an income (after tax) of **£400.00–500.00** per person per week.

7 Income and earnings which give a weekly income (after tax of more than **£600.00** per person per week.

TABLE 3.9 *Suggestion boxes — Wants or Needs?*

Step Four

Follow this exercise up by researching the following questions:

1 What is the **average annual income**, before tax, of:
- a single employed man in his twenties in the U.K.?
- a single employed women in her twenties in the U.K.?
- a married man in employment?
- a married women in employment?

For each of the categories above, work out how much the **annual** income works out at **per week.**

2 What income from **social security** could an unemployed man or woman in their twenties expect to receive per week in the U.K. today?

3 What income from **social security** could a married couple with two children under sixteen expect to receive per week in the U.K. today?

4 What does the **current state pension** pay, per week, to:
- a single man or woman?
- a married couple?

Research Round-Up

Sociologists study why people, in the societies to which they belong, behave and think in the ways they do. **Economists** study the ways in which the resources of a society (money, wealth, income) are distributed, used and controlled. Part of their work involves carrying out **research** into how social and economic factors can affect aspects of personal development such as health, education, employment opportunities and self–concept or self–esteem. **Some** examples of this research and the ideas and theories which arise form it are given here. However, students may find the table on page 262 useful in helping them find and organise more examples of the links between personal development and social and economic influences. Look out for the 'Other issues to explore…' sections.

Social factors

GENDER

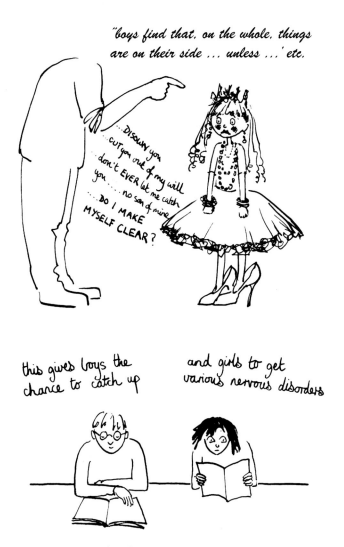

FIGURES 3.22 & 3.23 *Cartoons: Jacky Fleming.*

262 INTERMEDIATE Ⓖ Ⓝ Ⓥ Ⓠ HEALTH AND SOCIAL CARE

Each of us has a particular anatomical (bodily) sex. We are male or female. However, the behaviour and attitudes expected of men and women can vary between societies or between groups of people within a society. For example, while men in France, Italy and some South American countries can kiss or embrace each other because it is seen as normal behaviour, most men in the U.K. (according to a NOP survey in 2000) would rather shake another man's hand than kiss him and would only kiss a man if they were drunk or celebrating a sporting triumph. These expectations of male or female behaviour form our ideas of masculinity and femininity. There is an interesting debate about how much our gender roles are influenced by genetic and biological factors and how much by social and economic factors. Whatever the links between 'nature' and 'nurture' may be, we begin in childhood, to learn that boys and girls are different and that our society expects males and females to do different things and behave in different ways.

You can investigate the extent to which gender roles influence men and women's lives (and how they might be changing) by carrying out research into the kinds of social trends illustrated in Table 3.10 below. This table is not complete. There are many more aspects of the influence of gender on health, self–esteem, education and employment which could be explored and some suggestions for what to research are given below the table. You could also use this type of table to collect information about the other social and economic factors discussed below.

ASPECT OF PERSONAL DEVELOPMENT	SOCIAL FACTOR	POSITIVE INFLUENCES?	NEGATIVE INFLUENCES?
Health	Gender	Women live five years longer, on average, than men. Men are much more likely than women to take vigorous exercise for at least 20 minutes three times a week. Women's diets are healthier. They eat more fruit and are less likely to eat chocolate. Fewer women than men are overweight.	More women than men are obese or underweight.
Self–esteem	Gender	Boys with close and warm relationships with their mothers tend to have higher self–esteem.	Girls and women are more likely than boys and men to experience depression and eating disorders such as anorexia nervosa.

ASPECT OF PERSONAL DEVELOPMENT	SOCIAL FACTOR	POSITIVE INFLUENCES?	POSITIVE INFLUENCES?
Self-esteem (continued)			Girls worry more than boys about almost everything, and their levels of anxiety contribute to a loss of self-esteem. Their main worry is their appearance. Research published in 1998 by the Health Education authority found a marked association between worrying and 'substance abuse' — smoking, alcohol and drugs.
Education	Gender	Girls arrive in primary school with a much stronger grasp, on average, of the alphabet, numbers and most other aspects of learning, including social development.	Working–class boys drastically outnumber girls in schools and special units for children with learning and emotional social difficulties.
		Ten per cent more girls than boys get five GCSEs. There was a 66% rise in female undergraduates between 1990–91 and 1995–96.	Boys are more likely than girls to truant and be expelled from school.
Employment	Gender	Men outnumber women in permanent employment. Women are more likely to work 'flexitime' and less likely to be long–term unemployed than men. They form the majority of workers in health, education and public administration. More than two–thirds of women return to work within 9–11 months of giving birth.	Men are more likely than women to work very long paid hours with one in five working more than 50 hours a week. Women however, are still more likely to do the majority of the household tasks and child care. In paid employment women still earn, on average, nearly twenty per cent less than men.

TABLE 3.10 *Researching the effect of gender on personal development.*

Other issues to explore

1 Which illnesses are women more likely to develop than men?
2 Women form the majority of carers for elderly and/or disabled relatives. Why is this?

Family and friends

Today, the two–parent, 1.7 children family, although still fairly common, is not the only type of family young people in the UK will experience. The UK has the highest marriage rate and the second highest divorce and remarriage rate in Europe. This, coupled with the increase in young, single parenthood, means Britain is a nation with an increasing supply of step, half– and 'almost' relatives. Since the 1970s, these changes have meant that individuals, as they move through the various stages of their lives (childhood, young adulthood, adulthood, old age) may experience differing forms of the family, of which the two parent, 'nuclear family' may be only one.

Our families and friends, have, however, a very strong influence on our lives. For example, research by the Joseph Rowntree Foundation published in 1998 suggested that step–parents are more likely than other parents to be unhappy and to be poorer financially with lower–status jobs and less general support and help from the wider society.

Families have to support young people in the move from school to work for much longer periods than they did thirty or forty years ago. One in three 18 year olds now goes on to higher education, three times as many as in 1970. However, students are far worse–off money–wise than they were; increased drop–out rates from courses are mainly associated with financial difficulties. At the same time, the number of young people in work has fallen from 6.5 million in 1985 to under 4 million in 1997. There are few other options for young people besides education and training opportunities. More jobs require qualifications. It takes much longer for young people to qualify, gain employment and save enough money to move away from their parent's home and set up home separately. All these pressures can put strains on family relationships.

Other issues to explore

1 What is the impact of divorce and separation on children affected?
2 What role do families play in the socialisation of young children?

Age–groups

Groups of people of similar ages may be expected to share similar status and roles in society. For example, while in general people are living longer these days, the period of 'old age' is often viewed negatively rather than positively. Old people are stereotyped as 'out of touch', 'over the hill' and are often discriminated against in employment and access to services. However, research is showing that those people who follow advice to avoid smoking and excessive alcohol consumption, eat a low–fat diet high in fruit and vegetables and low in animal products and keep fit and active, are much more likely to enjoy a happy and fulfiling old age. Moreover, the 'use it or lose it' idea seems also to apply to our brain cells. A good early education and an interest in 'lifelong learning', keeps our bodies producing new connections between the nerve cells in the brain. This may help to stave off dementia and memory impairment in old age.

Other issues to explore

The period of 'adolescence' and the idea of 'youth culture'. How do relationships change during this period? What social and economic factors might influence personal development during this period? What ceremonies or traditions do different societies use to mark the passage from childhood to adolescence and from adolescence to adulthood?

Culture and ethnicity

Culture refers to the way of life of a society, its language, customs, dress, symbols and traditions. Ethnicity means the shared identity which arises from a common culture, religion or tradition. There is a multitude of ways in which these factors may influence health, education, employment prospects, self–concept and self–esteem.

One issue, the link between ethnicity and self–concept, will be explored here. In 2001 the national, ten–yearly Census will include the question "what is your ethnic group?". Possible answers will include white, Black Caribbean, white and black African, white and black Asian and, for the first time, a new 'mixed' category, with space to elaborate.

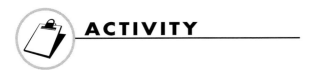 **ACTIVITY**

Questions to discuss.

1 **What would you tick?**
2 **Why do you think the Census includes a question on ethnic group?**
3 **Do you see yourself as belonging to a particular ethnic group?**
4 **What does 'ethnicity' mean to you? What might it mean to have a 'black 'identity or a 'white' identity?**
5 **Do you think it is possible to separate people into ethnic categories? Why or why not?**
6 **How important are factors such as skin colour, a shared culture or religion in our view of ourselves? Are other aspects of our tastes, lifestyles, beliefs and attitudes more or less important?**

Other issues to explore

Britain is a multicultural society. How might different cultural expectations and traditions affect people' s health, education and employment prospects? For example, there are different cultural traditions about:

- The use of body language;
- Touch (e.g. feelings about physical examinations);
- The distance between individuals (e.g. attitudes towards privacy);
- Accepted forms of address and respect;
- Diet;

- Religious practices (such as circumcision);
- Preferences for types of medical treatment;
- Birth and death customs;
- Sexual attitudes and roles;
- Washing and personal hygiene routines.

Discrimination and stereotyping

Discrimination means treating a person or group of people unfairly, usually because of a negative view of some or all of their characteristics. Stereotyping occurs where all members of group are viewed in the same, often simplified way. For example, 'all women drivers are hopeless' or 'young people today are irresponsible and lazy' are stereotyped views of those groups. Stereotypes are learnt by children from their parents and communities and from the culture which they grow up in, including the mass media.

The effects of discrimination can be both long term, resulting in patterns of disadvantage for whole groups in the population, and short term, resulting in immediate feelings of anger and/or loss of self–esteem and self–confidence. Three well–researched and, unfortunately all too common forms of discrimination in the U.K. are **racial and sexual discrimination** and **discrimination against people with disabilities**.

However, there are some other groups of people in society who may also suffer loss of self–esteem, poor health and reduced education and employment opportunities. For example, those with **mental health problems** may suffer particularly acutely:

- 1 in 7 people has a mental health problem in the U.K.
- Up to 1 in 4 children and young people have experienced depression and eating disorders and have been involved in substance misuse, deliberate self–harm and attempted suicide.
- An estimated 120,000 people a year are admitted to hospital in England and Wales following an episode of deliberate self–harm.
- The number of attempted suicides is estimated to be ten times the number of completed suicides.
- Diagnosed depression is twice as common in women as in men.

People experiencing mental health problems can be discriminated against in various ways. They are often seen or stereotyped as 'dangerous'. They receive a high level of verbal and physical abuse from others. They can be discriminated against when trying to find or stay in work, when trying to gain medical or welfare services or when trying to find a place to live.

Other issues to explore

1   Racial discrimination and its effects on health, education, employment and self–concept.
2   Sexual discrimination and its effects on health, education, employment and self–concept.
3   Discrimination against people with disabilities and its effects as above.

Isolation and social exclusion

Isolation means lack of membership of or rejection from certain groups in society. Most people can understand or imagine some of the effects this can have on health and self–esteem. For many children, their first unwelcome experience of this process is through being bullied or excluded from friendship groups at school.

Social exclusion refers to what can happen when people or areas suffer from a **combination** of linked problems such as unemployment, poor skills, low incomes, poor housing, high crime rates, bad health, poverty and family breakdown. Research has shown that there are 3000 neighbourhoods in England alone with deep–seated problems of run–down or derelict housing. The Independent Inquiry into Health Inequalities 1999 found that Britain is now the most unequal country in the world after the US, in terms of the gap between rich and the poor, which is wider than at any time since the second world war. A quarter of all children in Britain under 11 live in families on income support. Children from disadvantaged family backgrounds are more likely to be in disadvantaged socio–economic positions in later life and are likely to have worse health and survival rates.

Other issues to explore

- Bullying in schools.
- Exclusion from school and its effects on educational achievement.
- Poverty and disadvantage in Britain today.

ACCESS TO SERVICES

Health services

In the U.K. the National Health Service was set up to provide health care for all. However, people do not have equal access to healthcare services. Some of the social and economic factors already discussed can make a difference to the type of treatment or service people receive and may therefore affect their health, employment prospects and view of themselves For instance:

- People with physical disabilities, the elderly or people with young children may find it difficult to manage the journey to hospitals or clinics. If they are also living in poverty, they may be unable to pay transport costs, to arrange the necessary child care to allow them to visit a doctor or hospital or attend a clinic. While 11% of the population pays for private health insurance which gives them access to private health treatment, others have to wait up to four days for an appointment with their G.P. or months for a hospital operation.

- NHS rules mean that it is difficult for the homeless to register with a G.P. because they do not have a postal address, although some doctors do register homeless people by giving the surgery address on the form required. The fact that the homeless are up to 25 times more likely to die early than the average citizen supports the view that it is the most vulnerable groups that have the lease access to health care.

- In rural areas, poor public transport may put some people off visiting health professionals.

- Certain ethnic groups are less likely to use health services and, even when they do so, they may find that language difficulties prevent them from obtaining the most effective health care.
- Men appear to be less willing to use preventative health care than women.
- The elderly are sometimes discriminated against in access to health care and health treatments.
- The availability of health care varies throughout the country. For example, waiting times for hospital treatment, the drugs prescribed; and the availability of expertise and a specialist treatment centre for conditions such as cancer differs from one area to another.

Education

In August 1998, figures supplied by the major examining boards in this country showed that at GCSE level, 2.3% of young people sitting GCSEs received no award whatsoever. About 183,000 young people left school in the previous year with no GCSEs at all. Young people from poorer areas of the country were much more likely to leave school with fewer qualifications and much less likely to go on to higher education. Those young people are likely to suffer greater job insecurity, poorer working conditions, industrial injury and more overall experience of unemployment and low income in their lives. Although there are exceptions, for most people their schooling affects their future economic status and income.

Other issues to explore

1   What are the advantages (and disadvantages?) of access to pre–school or nursery education? How does provision vary between different parts of the country?
2   How could services for pregnant mothers and new parents be improved?

Housing

People who live in unhealthy homes usually suffer from other forms of social and economic disadvantage, so it becomes difficult to disentangle the effect of housing conditions on development from other factors. Moreover, there may be links between housing conditions and health not necessarily connected to poverty. For example, it has been suggested that the trend towards centrally heated homes with fitted carpets has increased the likelihood of allergies (and possibly asthma) resulting from 'dust mites'.

ENVIRONMENTAL INFLUENCES

See also p 176. Pollution of the environment can have a significant effect on our health, growth and personal development.

Water Pollution

Humans need water for a wide variety of uses. It must be clear and not contaminated with pollutants, in order to prevent infectious diseases and poisoning.

Toxic chemicals in industrial, agricultural and domestic waste are common pollutants of water. Purification is carried out before water is used, but although the treatment can remove organic waste and some bacterial contamination, it cannot cope with heavy chemical pollution. Examples of chemical pollutants in water include the following:

- Lead is taken into humans via air, food and water. It concentrates in the liver, kidney and bones. There is evidence that in children it can cause mental retardation.
- Nitrates enter water from fertilisers which are leached out of soil.

Air pollution

Children are particularly susceptible to air pollution, partly because of their large lung surface area and body volume ratio, which is a factor of their small size.

Asthma is a condition thought largely to result from air pollution, particularly of traffic emissions. Some asthma facts:

- Asthma affects 1 in 7 children.
- It is the most important cause of emergency hospital admissions.
- Respiratory diseases account for a third of children's G.P. visits.
- Asthma accounts for 1 in 20 childhood deaths.
- Hospital admission for asthma have increased 13-fold since the early 1960s.

Lead is the most serious heavy–metal pollutant in the atmosphere. The lead in car exhaust fumes accounts for about 80%, with the remainder coming from industrial processes. Even very low levels of lead in the blood can affect cognitive development and behaviour, with potentially long–term effects, and higher levels result in damage to the kidneys, liver and reproductive system. Growth can be affected.

Traffic in Britain is predicted to rise by 87% over the next 30 years. While vehicles are producing fewer harmful emissions, there will be more of them and people will travel longer distances. Diesel–fuelled vehicles, which produce 100% more poisonous emissions than petrol engines, are likely to triple over the next ten years.

Noise pollution

Noise is defined as unwanted sound. Because it can be a health hazard, it can be considered as a form of pollution. Noise maps produced by the Council for the Protection of Rural England show that there are very few tranquil areas remaining in England. With forecasts of huge traffic increases in the next twenty years, noise levels are set to increase further.

Sounds above about 90dB (decibels) can damage hearing. If exposure is over a long period, this damage can be permanent.

Other issues to explore

1   What risks to the environment and the child may be caused by the use of disposable nappies for babies and toddlers? Are reusable 'Terry' nappies more environmentally friendly?

2 Is the health of non–smokers at risk if they share the same environment as smokers? Should smoking be banned in all public and workplaces? What are the risks of 'passive' smoking?

Economic factors

If you have tried out the 'Wants and Needs' game on p 259 you will have realised that there is no easy way to work out how much money, income or wealth is needed for a healthy and happy life. Many people's main **income** is wages from employment, but other sources of income include benefits, pensions, interest from savings and dividends from shares. **Wealth** means something slightly different from income because it refers to the total value of the possessions held by an individual (or society). Some possessions, such as a small business, factory or a farm, can be a source of income for the people they belong to.

In Britain wealth is very unevenly divided among the population. Half the population shares between them only 7% of the total marketable wealth of the country in 1996; the other half of the population owns 93% of the total wealth of the country. In 1997–8, 30% of households had no savings at all. The gap between the rich and poor can also be measured by how much income people receive. In 1998 the proportion of people living on an income of less than half the average income in Britain (which is generally seen as an indication of living in **poverty**) was 24% of the population.

Just as it is very difficult to work out the differences between 'wants' and 'needs', so it is difficult to define and measure poverty. Poverty is a state in which, for an individual or a family, there is either a lack of resources sufficient to maintain a healthy existence (absolute poverty) or a lack of resources sufficient to achieve a standard of living considered acceptable in that particular society (relative poverty). Nevertheless, there are clear links between income and wealth and health, education, employment and self–esteem. These are discussed in more detail in Chapter 2, p 182.

Self–concept and self–esteem

Children develop a sense of identity and a self–concept during the first year of life. A self–concept is one's idea or image of oneself, and it involves an awareness of a sense of separateness from others and an increasing sense of self–awareness. The infant begins to be able to recognise 'particular others' and to search for them when they disappear from view. For most children, the realisation that they are a separate being from others occurs during the first two or three months of life.

Examples: When a baby touches a mobile, it moves; when they cry, someone responds; when they close their eyes, the world becomes dark.

The next stage in the development of self–concept is for the child to realise that not only do they exist separately from others but they have characteristics that form a '**me**'.

Example: The child understands that they have a name, gender and — later — other qualities such as clumsiness, shyness or adventurousness.

A study in self–awareness — The 'Mirror' Technique

Lewis and Brooks–Gunn (1979) placed infants aged between 9 and 12 months in front of a mirror. After allowing the infants time for free exploration — during which they typically looked at their own reflected images or tried to interact with the infant in the mirror — the experimenter secretly put a spot of rouge on the infant's nose and then let them look again in the mirror. The crucial test of self–awareness was whether the infant would reach for the spot on their own nose and not the nose on the face in the mirror. None of the infants aged 9–12 months touched their own noses (see Figure 3.24). When the experiment was repeated with infants aged 21 months, 75% of the infants touched their own noses.

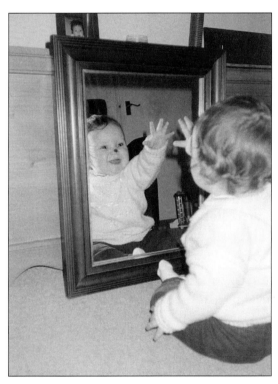

FIGURE 3.24 *At 9 months old, Emily reaches for the red spot on the face in the mirror, rather than her own face.*

THE DEVELOPMENT OF THE SELF–CONCEPT

Several factors play an important part in the development of a self–concept.

1   **How other people treat and react to us can affect how we see ourselves**. If we are consistently encouraged and praised for something we do, we may be more likely to begin to see ourselves as 'good' at that activity. A child who is repeatedly described by his parents as 'very shy' or 'very lazy' may begin to see himself in that way. It may become part of the way the child describes himself.

CHILDREN LEARN WHAT THEY LIVE

If children live with criticism, they learn to condemn.
If children live with hostility, they learn to fight.
If children live with fear, they learn to be apprehensive.
If children live with pity, they learn to feel sorry for themselves.
If children live with ridicule, they learn to feel shy.
If children live with jealousy, they learn to feel envy.
If children live with encouragement, they learn confidence.
If children live with tolerance, they learn patience.
If children live with praise, they learn appreciation.
If children live with acceptance, they learn to love.
If children live with approval, they learn to like themselves.
If children live with recognition, they learn it is good to have a goal.
If children live with sharing, they learn generosity.
If children live with honesty, they learn truthfulness.
If children live with fairness, they learn justice.
If children live with kindness and consideration, they learn respect.
If children live with security, they learnt to have faith in themselves and in those about them.
If children live with friendliness, they learn the world is a nice place in which to live.

— Dorothy Law Nolte

FIGURE 3.25 *Poem A child by Dorothy Law Nolte*

2 **How we compare ourselves with others can affect how we see ourselves**. For example, girls' worries about their body shape may be influenced by super-thin models and actresses used in advertising and some TV series such as 'Friends.'

3 **The social roles we play (parent, brother, teacher, worker, friend) affect our view of ourselves**. As we grow older and experience more of these roles, we tend to describe ourselves in terms of these roles.

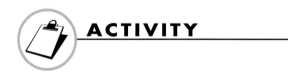

ACTIVITY

1 **Ask a group of ten or more people of different ages to describe themselves in twenty statements. Make sure you note the age of each person you ask to complete this activity.**

2 **Sort the types of statements each person makes into categories (e.g. statements about physical appearance, statements about personality or character, or statements about feelings, statements about likes and dislikes, statements about social roles or beliefs). Note how many of each type of statement is made by the people you ask. Is there a difference between the kinds of statements made by younger and older people?**

4 **The way in which we try to be like or identify with other people affects our view of ourselves.** We can want to identify ourselves with other people and 'be like them' for many

reasons, including the need for acceptance or status within a group or because we admire certain qualities in other people. In our 'success-oriented' culture there may also be pressures to try to be like those considered to be most successful in the society.

5 **The way in which we acquire a gender identity will have a significant affect on our view of ourselves.**

Developing self-esteem

Self-esteem is the regard people have of themselves. Our feelings of self-worth or self-esteem can strongly influence our moods and our behaviour. Sometimes we can hold very different views of ourselves to the views others hold of us. Even before a child can understand spoken words, parents and caregivers can show approval, disappointment, anger or pleasure by the tone of their voice, their facial expressions and general body language. Having a high self-esteem increases self-confidence and may make it possible for individuals to cope more easily with conflict and aggression than those with low self-esteem.

- High self-esteem during childhood has been linked with contentment and happiness in later life.
- Low self-esteem during childhood has been linked to anxiety, depression and maladjustment both in school and in social relationships.

Developing positive self-esteem goes hand in hand with **emotional literacy**, that is, understanding our feelings and emotions, the effect of other people's behaviour on us and our behaviour on others and being able to make positive changes when we want to.

Life-changes

During a person's lifetime, events can happen which will change their life. These changes can be predictable or unpredictable and often differ, in their effect, from the gradual and less remarkable everyday growth and development which occurs. Figure 3.26 illustrates some of these life-changing events.

LIFE CHANGES	
changes in location Moving house/job/school leaving home moving to another country or part of a country holidays retirement	changes in relationships marriage and cohabitation divorce or separation birth of a sibling death of a relative or friend- bereavement
changes in society war changes in the workplace advances in technology the 24-hour society being a victim of crime	physical changes puberty injury/accident/disability pregnancy and childbirth long-term illness

FIGURE 3.26 *Life-changes.*

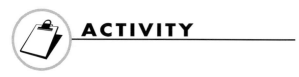

ACTIVITY

Use Figure 3.26 to discuss the possible effects of each group of life–changes described.

1 Which life–events may be more predictable than others?
2 What difference does it make if we can anticipate some of the major life–events we experience?
3 What might be some of the positive and negative effects of major life–changes?
4 Can we experience too many changes in our lifetimes? Is it better to experience few or many changes in our lives? Is their any evidence that 'overall life stress' is increasing?
5 Which life–changes might lead to the most anxiety and worry? Do men and women react differently to different life–changes?
6 In what different ways do people cope with life–changes?
7 What major changes have you and your family had to cope with in your life? If you had to make a list of the most significant events in your life, what would you include and why?

Types of support

People have different ways of coping with changes in their lives. As we have seen in this chapter, everyone has needs which must be met to achieve health and well–being. However, patients and clients in care settings may not be able to meet these needs themselves and may need support. This is especially the case when people go through difficult and traumatic life–changes. In this section of the chapter you should try to apply what you have learnt about the four areas of human need to thinking about the kind of support people may need.

As discussed on p 162 the simplest ways to think about needs is to consider the:

Physical
Intellectual
Emotional
Social needs of an individual

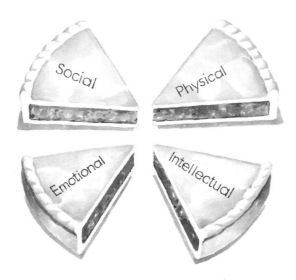

PHYSICAL NEEDS

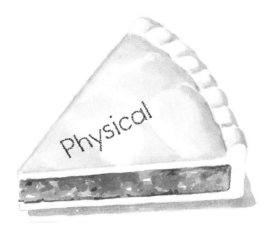

Physical needs include the need for food, drink, warmth, exercise, and freedom or relief from pain and discomfort.

The following two case studies illustrate examples of physical needs which must be met.

● *CASE STUDY* ● *CASE STUDY* ● *CASE STUDY* ● *CASE STUDY* ● *CASE STUDY* ● *CASE STUDY* ●

Mr. Brown

Mr Brown (80) is staying in the rehabilitation unit of his local hospital before he moves back home. He had a fall and broke his femur (thigh bone). Before he goes home the Occupational Therapist will assess his walking and mobility. He will also be assessed to see if he can make himself a drink and prepare simple food. If necessary, he will have additional support from a shopping service, home help and meals on wheels, to make sure his physical needs are met. When he leaves the rehabilitation unit, he will be given his prescriptions, including painkillers for the pain in his leg. Under current government policy, all people of retirement age are entitled to a winter heating payment (currently £150.00) to ensure that they can pay their fuel bills and keep warm in winter.

Our physical needs change during our life. In the early years, we depend on others to feed, clothe and support us. If we become ill, we may rely on other people. In order to keep health, we need to make sure our physical needs are met. If we are working in health and social care, we need to make sure that our clients or patients have their physical needs met.

● *CASE STUDY* ● *CASE STUDY* ● *CASE STUDY* ● *CASE STUDY* ● *CASE STUDY* ● *CASE STUDY* ●

Ann's story

"I was visiting my mother in a busy surgical ward at the local hospital. Because the staff were so busy, I used to help my mother at meal times, but I noticed that nurses tended to put meal trays down in front of patients and not wait to see if they could manage. There was another woman on the ward with a drip in her arm who had great difficulty managing. I was worried that she was not eating enough, but I felt awkward saying anything to the nurses.

What do you think I should have done?"

INTELLECTUAL NEEDS

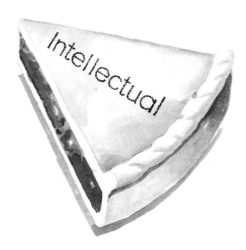

Intellectual needs are about having enough mental stimulation in order to keep the mind active and interested in life, through doing things such as reading, watching television, going to the cinema, playing games and doing crosswords. If a person is physically fit, they are able to do many things but the physically disabled and people with learning difficulties often find that access to many of these activities can be difficult, either because of the nature of their disability or because the society they live in does not make it easy for people with disabilities to play a full part. Contrast the attitudes towards disability expressed in Figures 3.27 and 3.28 below.

The disability discrimination act passed last month hasn't made life any easier for **Jane Parkinson** and her son, who uses a wheelchair

Our shrinking world

Part III of the new disability discrimination act states that buildings should provide a "reasonable alternative method" of access for a disabled person where a physical feature makes it difficult.

In what circumstances is it reasonable to expect an alternative? Most of my friends' houses are becoming inaccessible to us. So are the local post office and chemist. The main Oxford cinema, the Odeon, usually shows the latest children's blockbusters upstairs at inaccessible screen two; the Oxford museum is inaccessible due to its age; and the little science museum, CurioXity, is up a steep narrow staircase in the old fire station. Stiles and kissing gates prohibit country walks around Oxfordshire.

I am beginning to find it scary. I have always been lucky enough to be able-bodied and fit but my son, Alasdair, is severely physically disabled and if he can't go somewhere, I can't either. Neither can our friends when they are with us. Previously familiar environments present closed doors, secret places accessible only to the able-bodied.

The world is closing down around us and odd other worlds are opening up: now we take extremely long circuitous routes down thoughtfully provided slopes, sometimes not leading directly to where we wanted to go. We often end up in unexpected places – the gangway to a lift that led through the insalubrious kitchens of a service station on the M1; at Didcot railway station in an old-fashioned clangy lift full of

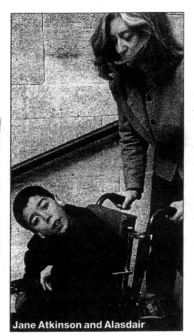

Jane Atkinson and Alasdair

postbags; in a bookshop squeezed next to a person-high stack of boxes of books. Cinemas and theatres everywhere are very fond of telling us sanctimoniously that we are a fire hazard, or leading us

proudly to the designated wheelchair space behind a pillar.

The manager of a country pub full of American tourists tried to tell me that the building was much too old to make any changes that might make it accessible to wheelchair-users. When I pointed out that the spacious loos could easily be adapted, he admitted: "We don't really need the custom."

At our local school my son is unable to join his peers in their move up to the next class until the Oxford education authority decides whether it can and will provide the funds for a stairlift.

Why should it, you may ask – why can't he just go to a school that is on one level? Indeed. And we shall take all future holidays in Milton Keynes and choose only friends who live in ground floor flats.

FIGURE 3.27 *Our shrinking world.*

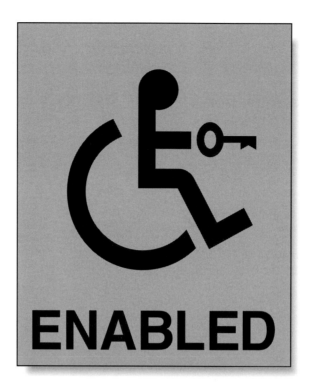

For the past fifty years Leonard Cheshire has enabled thousands
of disabled people to lead more fulfilling lives. Making it possible
for them to live in their own homes is just one of the
ways we have achieved this.

Leonard Cheshire creates opportunity

This is an opportunity for you to help. Please make a donation today
and help us prove that a disability doesn't have to be a handicap.

Creating opportunities with disabled people

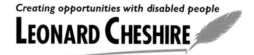

FIGURE 3.28 *Enabled.*

● CASE STUDY ● CASE STUDY ● CASE STUDY ● CASE STUDY ● CASE STUDY ● CASE STUDY ●

Henry

Henry is 26. He lives in a small private residential home for people with learning difficulties. There are 8 residents in the home, 4 men and 4 women. Although Henry has Downs Syndrome, he has good communication skills and he is encouraged to be independent. In his room he has a sound system he is proud of, and a television, although he prefers to watch T.V. in the lounge with the other residents. Every weekday he attends the training centre where he works, packing plastic cutlery. He enjoys this. Every Saturday he goes shopping for magazines and CDs in the local shopping centre. He visits the library and goes to the pub.

As you can see from this case study, everyone has intellectual needs. This does not mean we have to be 'brainy' but we all need interests to keep our minds active. In care work, you need to consider how the intellectual needs of your clients and patients may be met. This could be through a range of activities from art and crafts to the use of computers which have special applications for people with disabilities.

EMOTIONAL NEEDS

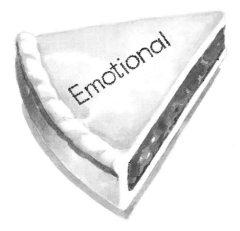

Emotional needs are met by having a sense of belonging, helping people to feel secure and safe. We all need to feel accepted and valued by others and to feel part of a group. For some people these needs may he met by being in family or being part of a group of close friends.

● *CASE STUDY* ● *CASE STUDY* ● *CASE STUDY* ● *CASE STUDY* ● *CASE STUDY* ● *CASE STUDY* ●

Susan

Susan (18) has just started her Diploma in nursing course. Although Susan has always lived in Southampton, she decided she wanted to do her course in London. She had visited London several times. All her friends are working or studying in different parts of the country.

Susan is lucky as the School of Nursing has provided accommodation for the students, so she is sharing a house with several people on her course. She finds it easy to make friends as all the students are hoping to follow a career in ursine and seem to have similar interests. Within a few weeks she has formed a circle of friends to go out with, and two special friends she can talk to about anything.

Emotional needs are very important throughout life. Career changes, moving house and the changes which occur at different life–stages may mean that the people we once relied on for support are no longer around, so we need to develop new sources of emotional support. During major life changes, such as severe illness or bereavement, we need the support of professionals, such as doctors, psychologists or counsellors. We need to ensure that our emotional needs are met, in order for us to achieve health and well–being.

SOCIAL NEEDS

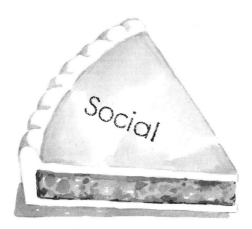

Social needs are about forming relationships with other people, living and working together. Many people will have their social needs met through friends and colleagues at school, college and work. Others will rely more on their family, or organised groups such as clubs.

● *CASE STUDY* ● *CASE STUDY* ● *CASE STUDY* ● *CASE STUDY* ● *CASE STUDY* ● *CASE STUDY* ●

Vikram

Vikram (60) is a retired businessman. He had to retire early because of a heart condition. He worked long hours and 'lived for his work'. When he retired he found he became very depressed because all the social contacts he had were related to his work. He still attended meetings of the Rotary Club, and helped with fund raising activities for local charities, but he felt that his skills were not being fully used, and he wanted to meet more people.

He lives in a London borough in which is very ethnically mixed and houses many refugees. He joined several local voluntary groups assisting refugees, setting up day centres and advising people of their rights. He helped people apply for jobs and benefits, and acted as translator for some groups. He now feels that he is well known in the community, and is using his skills to help others.

As we can see from all the case studies above, physical, intellectual, emotional and social needs are all closely inter–linked. Vikram has built up a social network to replace the one he lost at work, but the role he developed for himself in the community also fulfils his intellectual and emotional needs.

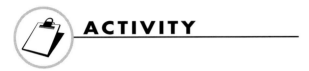

ACTIVITY

Read the case studies below about Beatrice and Imran

On two pieces of paper, one for Beatrice and one for Imran, draw four columns and label them with these headings:

Physical needs   Intellectual needs   Emotional needs   Social needs

Identify how each need, for Beatrice and Imran, is being met (for example, Beatrice's intellectual needs could be met by listening to the radio, so put radio in the appropriate column).

Case study Beatrice

Beatrice is an 88 year old grandmother. She enjoys pottering about in the garden, listening to the radio and reading the newspaper. Although she lives on her own, Beatrice is in regular contact with her son and married daughter, who both live nearby. Once a week, Beatrice attends the local Day Centre, where she has a meal and talks to some friends she has made. She can also book an appointment with the chiropodist or hairdresser while she is there. She attends the local diabetic clinic once a month, and uses Dial a Ride service to take her there and bring her home.

Case Study Imran

Imran is a lively 5 year old with cerebral palsy. He attends a special school each week day during term time. The school bus collects him each morning and brings him home. Imran tries to do as much as possible for himself, but he needs help with eating, drinking, washing and using the toilet. He can get around the house by holding on to things but he uses a wheelchair for longer distances. He has a computer in the living room and he enjoys playing games on that. At school he likes painting and swimming. He has a younger sister, Salma, who makes him laugh. His grandmother spends every evening with him, talking and reading. Imran's speech is affected by the cerebral palsy so strangers sometimes find it difficult to understand him. It also takes him longer to say things.

Beatrice lives independently and Imran is cared for by his family. If Beatrice and Imran had to live in residential care and be looked after by others, how could we be sure that their intellectual, emotional, social and physical needs were being met? Living in a different environment would have a very great impact on their lives.

Changing needs

As we go through life, our needs may change and the types of support we need may also alter. At each life stage individuals will have different needs which will be met in different ways. Support may be given by the following groups:

- **professionals** such as nurses, doctors, health visitors, occupational therapists, residential staff, counsellors and teachers.
- **voluntary workers**, such as volunteers at a day centre, crèche or youth club.
- **friends,** who can help with personal problems and major life–changes such as bereavement and divorce.
- **families**, who may be able to offer practical and emotional support.

ACTIVITY

1 Read the life history of Louise Phillips below.
2 Identify key changes in her life.
3 What types of support could have helped Louise? Remember the four types of need (PIES) when thinking about this.

··

● CASE STUDY ● CASE STUDY ● CASE STUDY ● CASE STUDY ● CASE STUDY ● CASE STUDY ●

Louise Phillips

Louise Phillips is 45. She was born in Manchester. She was an only child until her mother had another baby, a boy, when Louise was 10 years old. Louise went to a local play group, then to a nursery school At five, she attended the local infants school At 7 years old she was transferred to the junior school which was three miles from her home. She passed the 11+ examination and went to grammar school. She was the only girl from her class to get in. To reach her secondary school she had to take a train and a bus. Her parents were very proud of her but Louise found the work hard. She decided to take a secretarial course at the local college when she left school. When she finished this, she had several different jobs.

Louise married John when she was 21. Their first daughter Anne, was born when Louise was 22.

She still lived hear her mother, who helped her with the baby, but when Louise was 24, her mother died suddenly. When she was 26, John's firm moved to Reading and the family had to move to the south of the country. Louise found part–time secretarial work once her daughter Anne started school, but she had to give this up when she had her second baby, David, at the age of 32. John's job in Reading proved very stressful. By the time Louise was 38, her marriage had ended in divorce.

● CASE STUDY ● CASE STUDY ● CASE STUDY ● CASE STUDY ● CASE STUDY ● CASE STUDY ●

Louise Phillips (continued)

Louise decided she wanted to work in residential care, with a view to becoming a social worker. However, her daughter Anne, had started a university course and her son, David, was still at primary school when Louise was involved in a major car accident. She made a good recovery but could not work full–time any more. She is now investigating the possibility of taking a part–time degree course.

Looking at Louise's story, we can identify several key changes in her life when the support of professionals, voluntary workers and others could be helpful. For example:

Her first child is born:

This is a significant life–change. Professional support could be given by the midwife and health visitor. Voluntary support could be given through the National Childbirth Trust (NCT). Their helpers advise on breast feeding and others aspects of pregnancy, childbirth and child care. Family and friends could also support Louise, including young parents' groups, which could offer emotional and social support. Babysitters could give Louise the opportunity to go out or attend evening classes.

Her mother dies:

Loss and bereavement (see below), especially when it is sudden, means that many people will need emotional support. Professional support could include the G.P. and a counselling service. Counselling could be provided through the NHS or by private and voluntary agencies. The support of family and friends is very important at this time.

LOSS AND BEREAVEMENT

Most life–changes will have a positive and negative side. However, in this last section of the chapter, the impact of loss and bereavement and the types of support available to help people through this period in life will be discussed.

Loss is experienced in many ways, and does not necessarily involve the death of a loved one. For example, growing up involves the loss of all the infancy support networks; going to school involves temporary separation from parents; and changing school involves the loss of familiar surroundings. There are obviously corresponding 'gains' here as well; for example, the child will gain new friends and experiences with each change in circumstances. Other life events which involve loss are:

- new siblings (i.e. the loss of parental attention);
- the death of a sibling;
- bereavement, as grandparents grow older and die;
- the loss of a parent through separation, divorce or death;
- ending or changing relationships;
- unemployment (either the parent's, the sibling's or one's own);
- miscarriage, termination of pregnancy or stillbirth;
- disability (the loss of a sense of the future and of security);
- the birth of a baby with disability (parents may grieve for the 'normal' child they were expecting);
- caring for people with dementia or Alzheimer's disease.

Each loss may be viewed as a preparation for greater losses. How the individual reacts to the death of a loved one will depend on how they have experienced other losses, their personality, their religious and cultural background and the support available.

Grief

Grief is a normal and necessary response to the death of a loved one. It can be short-lived or it can last for a long time. Grief at the death of a husband, wife or child is likely to be the most difficult to get over. Grief can take the form of several clearly defined stages:

1 *shock and disbelief:* numbness and withdrawal from others enables the bereaved person to get through the funeral arrangements and family gatherings. This stage may last from three days to three months;

2 *denial:* this generally occurs within the first 4 days and can last minutes, hours or weeks. No loss is acknowledged; the bereaved person behaves as if the dead person were still there. Hallucinations are a common experience. These may consist of a sense of having seen or heard the dead person, or of having been aware of their presence.

3 *growing awareness:* some or all of the following emotions may be felt, and each conspires to make many people feel that they are abnormal to experience such harsh emotions:

   ➡ *yearning:* the urge to try to find a reason for the death;

   ➡ *anger:* directed against any or all of the following: the medical services; the person who caused the death, in the case of an accident; God, for allowing it to happen; the deceased, for abandoning them;

   ➡ *depression:* the pain of the loss is felt, often with feelings of a lack of self–esteem. Crying, or letting go, often helps to relieve the stress;

   ➡ *guilt:* this may be the guilt for the real or imagined negligence inflicted on the person who has just died; or the bereaved can feel guilty about their own feelings and inability to enjoy life;

   ➡ *anxiety:* often bordering on panic, as the full impact of the loss is realised. There is worry about the changes and the new responsibilities and future loneliness. There may even be thoughts of suicide.

4   *acceptance.* This usually occurs in the second year, after the death has been relived at the first anniversary. The bereaved person is then able to relearn the world and new situations without the deceased person.

Research has shown that counselling may help to reduce the damage to physical and emotional health which often follows the loss of a loved one. Most people come through the healing process of grief with the help of relatives and friends. Those who may be in particular need of help are often those:

● with little or no family support;

● with young children;

● who have shown particular distress or suicidal tendencies.

Bereavement counsellors try to establish a warm, trusting relationship with the bereaved person. This is done initially by listening with patience and sympathy; accepting tears as natural and even desirable. Bereavement counselling should not be undertaken by individuals working alone. The support of a group under professional guidance is vital, as close contact with intense grief can be very stressful and emotionally demanding.

Glossary

Adolescence — a time between childhood and adulthood when important physical changes occur, such as a sudden increase in growth and maturity.

Advocacy — where someone speaks on behalf of or represents the interests of someone else, particularly those who are less able to voice their views, because of, for example, learning difficulties, mental health problems or lack of knowledge or power. The advocate could be a professional volunteer or friend.

Ageism — discrimination based on age, meaning that a person is treated unfairly or differently because of their age.

Benefits Agency — the Agency within the Department of Social Security which is responsible for the assessment and payment of social security payments.

Bereavement — the loss of a loved one through death.

Carer — the person who takes responsibility for the care and support of a person who cannot fully support themselves.

Care plan — the plan of treatment and/or care agreed upon jointly by the service user and the named nurse or keyworker.

Childhood — a socially and physically defined stage in life describing the time before a person reaches adolescence or adulthood.

Census — the ten-yearly national Census in the UK is the largest possible survey of the population of the country and it is used to find out the size and composition of the population.

Cerebral palsy — a medical condition caused by damage or injury to the developing brain. This may occur during pregnancy, birth or in the early postnatal stages. There may be minor disabilities such as late walking and clumsiness or more severe disorders of posture, movement and co-ordination. There are different types of cerebral palsy depending on the part of the body affected. Children with cerebral palsy may suffer from movement which is jerky and uncontrolled.

Chiropodist — a qualified professional who has specialised in the treatment of feet and their associated disabilities and diseases.

Counselling — the process by which one person helps another person to help themselves. It is a way of relating and responding to another person so that they are helped to explore their thoughts, feelings and behaviour, in order to reach a clearer self-understanding.

Development — the process of acquiring new skills.

Downs Syndrome — a genetic condition caused by the presence of an extra chromosome; those with Downs' Syndrome have 47 chromosomes instead of the usual 46. About one baby in every 1000 has Down's Syndrome and they are usually born below average weight and length and have distinguishing features such as a face which appears flattened.

Discrimination — treating a person or group unfairly, usually because of a negative view of some or all of their characteristics.

District nurse — a qualified nurse who works closely with the GP and is employed by the Community Trust.

Domiciliary services — health and social care services that take place in the service user's home.

Economic factors — those factors in any situation which affect the ways in which people produce, obtain and uses the resources they require for things which are essential (such as food, clothing and housing) as well as non–essential items.

Emotional development — the development of self–image and identity, including the ways in which an individual makes sense of emotions in themselves, and of feelings towards other people.

Emotional literacy — the ability to understand and manage one's emotions and empathise with the feelings and perspectives of others.

Emotional needs — these include having a sense of belonging in society and may be met by being part of a family, group of friends or other social group.

Ethnicity — the sharing of a common history, set of customs an identity, as well as, in most cases, language and religion.

Fine manipulative skills — physical skills which involve small, intricate movements, such as writing or playing a musical instrument.

Gender — a term used to describe the social and cultural expectations of male or female behaviour. These expectations contribute to ideas about 'masculinity' and 'femininity', i.e. what behaviour and attitudes it is acceptable for men and women to display.

Gross motor skills — movements involving the use of large muscle groups, such as standing, running or jumping.

Growth — an increase in size and complexity.

Health Visitor — a registered nurse with additional training who works in the community to advise and support children under 8 and their families. The role has recently been expanded to include health promotion, including continence advice.

Hypothermia — a potentially life-threatening reduction of body temperature below the normal range. It is liable to occur in vulnerable clients such as elderly people and babies.

Income — a term generally used to mean the money which an individual, family or group receives over time. Many peoples' main income is wages from employment, but other sources of income include benefits, pensions, interest on savings and dividends from shares.

Identity — a person's understanding of his/her self in relation to other people and society.

Infancy — the stage in life from birth to one year.

Intellectual development — the development of perception, reasoning, understanding, and the acquisition of knowledge.

Intellectual needs — these include having enough mental stimulation to keep the mind active and interested in the wider world.

Isolation — lack of membership of or exclusion from social groups.

Key worker — a named person who ensures that a care plan is followed and care is giver to the client/patient. In health care, there will be a named nurse who is responsible for certain patients.

Learning disability — a lifelong condition which results from impairment to the brain before, during or after birth, or from genetic or chromosomal factors. An example is the condition called Down's Syndrome.

Life–changes — predictable or unpredictable but ***significant*** events in a person's life.

Menopause — the ending of menstruation, usually occurring naturally in women between 45 and 55 years of age. It marks the end of a woman's capacity for sexual reproduction.

Milestones (norms) — these are used to show what individuals can usually do at a particular age.

Occupational therapist — a trained professional who treats patients, clients and service users with temporary or permanent physical or learning disability or mental illness. The occupational therapist supports clients with different problems, such as psychological or physical illness, accident recovery or ageing.

Nitrates — potassium or sodium nitrates are commonly used as fertilisers in agricultural production. Using fertilisers can cause large amounts of nitrates to build up in the soil. Rainwater may then wash the nitrates into water supplies, rivers and the sea. High levels of nitrates in drinking water may cause illness. In seas, nitrates produce rapid growth of algae and other water plants that can badly affect fishing.

Passive smoking — the involuntary inhaling of smoke from others' cigarettes.

Peer pressure — the control exercised by a group of people sharing common characteristics (e.g. schoolchildren) to behave in the same way as others in the group. The most powerful form of peer pressure is usually the threat of exclusion from the group.

Physical needs — these include the need for food, drink, warmth, exercise and freedom or relief from pain and discomfort.

Poverty — a state in which, for an individual or a family, there is either a lack of resources sufficient to maintain a healthy existence (absolute poverty) or a lack of resources sufficient to achieve a standard of living considered acceptable in that particular society (relative poverty).

Puberty — the time at which secondary sexual characteristics (such as voice pitch and hair growth) start to develop.

Secondary sexual characteristics — genetically–determined characteristics that are not concerned with sexual reproduction, but are nonetheless different between sexes, such as body hair or voice pitch.

Self–concept or self–image — the way we view, understand and value ourselves.

Self–esteem — the value we place upon ourselves: our sense of self–worth.

Social development — the growth of the individual's relationships with others and the development of social skills.

Social factors — these describe the patterns in and expectations of social behaviour which may affect, for instance, people's health, their employment prospects, their level of education and their self–esteem.

Social exclusion — a term used to describe what can happen when people or areas suffer from a combination of linked problems such as unemployment, poor skills, low incomes, poor housing, high crime environments, bad health, poverty and family breakdown.

Social needs — these include the need to form relationships with other people, to live, work and enjoy leisure with other people.

Stereotyping — the process whereby groups or individuals are characterised in simplified and often negative terms, so that all members of a group are seen in one particular way.

Wealth — the total value of the possessions held by an individual or a society.

Youth culture — the idea that groups of young people in a society may share a similar way of life and adopt similar attitudes, tastes in music, clothes and leisure pursuits.

Answers

PHYSICAL GROWTH AND DEVELOPMENT

INFANCY–GROWTH
i) Between 4–5 months.

PUBERTY AND ADOLESCENCE; ADULTHOOD, OLD AGE

i)

Growth Motor Skills	Fine Manipulative Skills
Roller-Blading Skiing	Embroidery Playing the flute

Resources

Bruce, T. and Meggit C. (2000) *Child Care and Education*, Hodder and Stoughton, London. This is an excellent book which covers physical, intellectual, emotional and social development in babies and children.

Thomson, H.R. and Meggit C. (1996) *Human Growth and Development*, Hodder and Stoughton, London. This book covers physical, intellectual, emotional and social development throughout the life stages.

There are many other books, magazines and web sites which are aimed at parents and carers and which describe the development of babies and children. You will be able to find these in your local libraries, bookstores and newsagents. When using the Internet, you will find that the sites marked with an * below contain excellent LINKS to numerous other useful sites. Try using a search engine such as **www.google.com/** for reliable and quick reference to useful sites.

REFERENCES

Donald Acheson (Chair); The Independent Inquiry into Health Inequalities, Our Healthier Nation: Reducing Health Inequalities: An Action Report, (1999), Department of Health. Download this report in pdf at: **http://www.doh.gov.uk/pub.docs/doh/inequalities.pdf**

Elsa Ferri and Kate Smith, (1998), *Step-Parenting in the 1990s*, The Family Policy Studies Centre in association with the Joseph Rowntree Foundation.

Health Education Authority (Sept. 1998), *'The Impact of Discrimination on Mental and Emotional Well–Being,'* Surrey Social and Market Research, The University of Surrey, for the HEA

Jones, G., *Rites of Passage Rewritten*, TES Briefing Analysis, 11/6/98.

Lewis, M. and Brooks-Gunn, J., (1979) *Social Cognition and the Acquisition of Self*, New York: Plenum Press.

ORGANISATIONS

Joseph Rowntree Foundation
The Homestead
40 Water End
York
North Yorkshire YO30 6WP
Tel: +440(0) 1904629241
Website: **info@jrf.org.uk**

NOP Research Group
Website: **http://www.maires.co.uk/**

Office for National Statistics
Website: **http://www.ons.gov.uk**

Social Science Information Gateway (SOSIG)
Website: **http://www.sosig.ac.uk/**

National Asthma Campaign
Providence House
Providence Place
London N1 ONT
Tel: 0207 2262266

King's Fund
Website: **http://www.kingsfund.org.uk**

National Institute for Social Work
Website: **http://www.nisw.org.uk**

Government Information Service
Website: **www.open.gov.uk**

Schools Health Education Unit, Exeter University,
Renslade House
Bonhay Road
Exeter
Devon EX4 3AY
Website: **sheu@exeter.ac.uk**

Child Accident Prevention Trust
18-20 Farringdon Lane
London EC1R 3AU
Tel: 0171 6083828
Website: **http://childcare-now.co.uk/capt.html#top**

National Childbirth Trust
Alexandra House
Oldham Terrace
Acton
London W3 6NH
Tel: 0208 992 8637
Website: **http://www.nct-online.org./main.htm**

Council for the Protection of Rural England
Warwick House
25 Buckingham Palace Road
London SW1W OPP
Tel: +44(0) 2079766433
Website: **http://www.greenchannel.com/cpre**

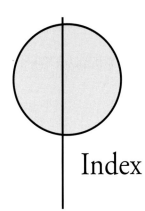

Index

A

abuse 106, 114
Access to Personal Files Act (1987)
    124
access to services 178, 267–8
Accident and Emergency 60, 62, 64,
    65, 103
action planning 8, 19, 22–3
activity theory 252, 254
acupuncture 65
addiction 188, 195
administration staff 99–100
adolescence 238–9, 265
    emotional and social development
    251–2
    growth 235, 238–9
    intellectual development 248–9
    physical development 244
adoption and fostering services 94,
    105, 106
adrenaline 203
adulthood
    emotional and social development
    252
    growth 235, 239
    intellectual development 248–9
    physical development 244
advocacy 146–7
age 77–8, 119–20, 158, 240, 264
AIDS/HIV 189, 206, 207, 208
alcohol abuse 190–4
alternative therapists 65
Alzheimers Disease 74–5, 127, 146–7
amphetamines 185
analysing 17, 18
anorexia nervosa 197–8, 199
ante natal services, access to 178
assessment vi
    clients' needs 41, 105
    course work 16
    external 28–30
    social services procedure 67, 68
    work-experience placement 46
assignments 17–18, 22–3, 43

asthma 181, 182, 215–17, 268, 269
audiology service 12

B

babies 170, 188–9, 236
bereavement 283–5
bibliographies, writing 27–8
block placements 42
BMI *see* Body Mass Index
body language 112–13, 121
Body Mass Index 214–15, 222
bottle feeding 170
brainstorming 17, 19
breast feeding 170, 171, 283
British Sign Language 139, 140
bulimia nervosa 198, 199
bullying 83, 267

C

caffeine 190, 191
cannabis 185
carbohydrates 165, 166, 167
care plans, for individuals 129–30
Care Value Base 118, 137
careers advice 150
carers 76–84
case-studies 2, 8, 16–28
charities 55, 73, 107–8
    Charities Digest, The 73
Charters of Rights 127–9
child psychiatrists 102
childhood
    emotional and social development
    251
    growth 235, 237–8
    intellectual development 247–8
    physical development 243–4
childminders 105
children 70, 98, 107, 170–1
Children Act (1989) 104–5
Children's Homes 106
children's nurse 98
chiropodists 92
chiropractics 65

Citizen's Advice Bureau 41, 42
class, and health 158, 181
classroom assistants 98
clinical psychologist 102
Code of Professional Conduct for
    Nurses 123, 126
Codes of Practice 126
communication skills 2, 28, 41
    alternative approaches to 137–47
    Alzheimers Disease and Dementia
    146–7
    barriers 110
    deaf blind 139, 143
    feedback 110
    hearing loss 139–43
    language barriers 137–9
    learning difficulties 145
    lip reading 139, 141–2
    listening skills 111–12
    non-verbal 112–16, 143
    questions, types of 109
    speaking difficulties 143–4
    on the telephone 115, 124–5
    verbal 108–10
    visual impairment 143
    written 116–18
community
    dental service 102
    homes 106
    paediatricians 102
    pharmacists 90
    psychiatric nurses 60, 85, 89
Community Mental Health Trusts 89,
    94
comparing 18
confidence 36
confidentiality 43, 44, 45, 122–5
CPNs *see* community, psychiatric
    nurses
culture, and personal development
    265–6

D
Data Protection Act (1984) 124
day care 67, 94, 96, 105
day care assistant, job description
    97–8
deaf blind people 139, 143
dementia 74, 146–7, 264
dental nurses 91
dentists 90–1
Department of Health 55, 56
dependence, on drugs 188, 195
depression 266, 284
describing 18
development, human 234–5
    emotional and social 249–54
    intellectual 245–9
    physical 241–5
    diaries 8, 45–6
diet 165–72, 181, 197–201, 204, 264
dignity, client's rights to 130–2
Disability Discrimination Act (1995)
    119, 277
disabled groups 1, 53, 94
    access to healthcare services 267
    discrimination 118, 266, 276–9
    exercise 175–6
    intellectual needs 276–9
    rights of 133
Disabled Students Allowance Scheme
    24, 53
discrimination 118–22, 266
discussing 18, 40
District Health Authorities 57–8, 90
district nurses 60, 89
divorce, effect on children 264
domiciliary care 67, 96
drugs 184–90, 190–6
dyslexia 1, 34, 53
dysphasia 143–4
dyspraxia 1, 34, 53

E
early years services 101–8
economic factors, in personal
    development 254–68, 270
economists 261
ecstasy (drug) 186
editing, assignments 25–6
education 65–6, 183, 254, 263, 268
Education Act (1993) 106
educational psychologists 102
emergency services 60, 62, 64, 65,
    103
emotions 161, 162–4, 203, 210, 234,
    273
empathy 211
employment 254, 263
empowerment 147, 278

enuresis clinic (bedwetting service)
    102
environmental influences 176, 268–70
equal opportunities policies 122
equipment and materials 9
ethnic groups 118, 121, 122, 265,
    268
evaluating 17, 18
evaluations 8, 23, 25, 46
examinations *see* tests, timed
exercise 173–6, 204, 205
explaining 18

F
families 70, 77, 264
Family Focus (charity) 107
family therapists 102
fats 165, 166, 167, 169, 171, 197
feedback 46
fibre 165, 166
field work 67, 95
fitness index 218–19, 222
foetal alcohol syndrome 192
folic acid 171–2
food 171, 181
fostering 94, 98, 105, 106
friends, and personal development
    264

G
gay men, discrimination 118
gender 158, 261–4, 268
Genito-Urinary Medicine 60, 207
glossaries 49–51, 151–3, 228, 286–9
Government Information Service 11
GPs 60, 86–7, 94, 129
grief 284–5
groups 37–40, 38–9
growth, stages in human 234–40
GUM *see* Genito-Urinary Medicine

H
hazards 134–5, 208–9
health
    aspects of 158–9, 161, 162–4
    education 177
    factors affecting 164–84, 255
    gender 262
    professional definitions 159–64
    promotion 210–11
    risks to 185–210
    subjective definitions 156–9
health and safety
    of clients 134–6
    in workplaces 45
Health and Social Care Boards
    (Northern Ireland) 57
Health Boards (Scotland) 55, 57

health care jobs 84–94
health centres, organisation of 100
health improvement plans 210–11
    producing 220–2
Health Improvement Programmes 57
health visitors 60, 88–9, 102
Healthier Schools Programme 102
hearing loss 139–43
height, and weight 212–15
Help the Aged 136
hepatitis 189
heroin 187
HImP *see* Health Improvement
    Programmes
HIV *see* AIDS/HIV
holiday care 107
home carer, job description 96
homeless, access to healthcare services
    267
homeopathy 65
hospital play specialists 104
hospitals 94
housing 180–2, 267, 268
hypothermia 181

I
ideas, organising and generating
    19–21
identifying 18
identity 136–7, 249
immunisation 101
'In the Hot Seat' (game) 258
income 177, 182–3, 255, 258–60,
    270
independence, client's rights to 132–4
infancy
    emotional and social development
        250–1
    growth 235–7
    intellectual development 246
    physical development 242
Informal Care 54, 55, 75, 76–84, 108
information technology 2, 28, 46, 48
inspections 105–6
intellectual development 161, 162–4,
    234
Internet, using 10–11
isolation 267

K
Key Skills Qualification 2, 28, 46–8
King's Fund 11

L
language barriers 137–9
learning difficulties, people with
    communicating with 145
    discrimination 118, 122

jobs working with 94
rights of 133
voluntary services for 70
learning styles 2, 3–4, 16
lesbians 118
libraries, using 2, 10, 11
life-changes 273–4, 281–3
lifestyle, and health 158, 210
linking words and phrases 23, 24
lip reading 139
listening skills 111–12
Local Authorities 57, 66, 126
locality 158, 268
log books 8, 45–6
loss 283–4

M
Makaton (language programme) 145
manipulative skills 241–2, 244–5
medicine, as a career 86–7
memory 2, 15, 28–9, 28–34, 29–34,
    30–1, 31–3, 249
Mencap 71–3
menopause 239
Mental Health Act (1960) 71
mental health problems, people with
    61, 70, 94, 118, 121, 266
methods of working 3–4
midwives, Code of Practice 126
milestones, in development 234
mind-mapping 14–15, 19, 20–1
minerals 165, 167
minimum wage 183
'mirror' technique 271
mirroring 113
Misuse of Drugs Act 184
Modernising Social Services (White
    Paper 1998) 67
monitoring work 23
mother and child support groups 107
motivation 8
motor skills 241–2, 244–5

N
National Childbirth Trust 283
National Drugs Helpline 187, 189
National Health Service see NHS
National Institute for Social Work 11
National Society for Mentally
    Handicapped Children and Adults
    see Mencap
National Society for the Prevention of
    Cruelty to Children 108
NCT see National Childbirth Trust
needs
    changing 281–3
    of clients 45
    emotional 279–80

intellectual 276–9
physical 275–6
social 280–1
versus wants 258–60, 270
New NHS, Modern Dependable
    (White Paper 1997) 55
NHS 11
    access to services 178, 267–8
    national organisation 55–7
    regional organisation 58
    staff numbers 84
NHS and Community Care Act
    (1990) 60, 69, 75
NHS Direct 60, 62–3, 90
Language line 138
NHS Internet Service 64
NHS Trusts 57, 60–1
    Community Mental Health Trusts
    89
    Community Trusts 61
    Hospital Trusts 60–1
    Mental Health Trusts 61, 94
NHS Walk In Centres 60, 64
nicotine 194–6
non-verbal communication 112–16,
    143
norms, in development 234
note-taking 2, 9–10, 12–14, 14–15
number, application of 2, 28, 48, 76
nursery nursing 98
nursing 87–9, 92–3, 93–4

O
obesity 197, 215
occupational therapists 67, 85, 99,
    105, 275
occupations
    and health 177–9, 209
    in health and social care 85–6
older people
    alcohol 192–3
    diet 172
    discrimination 118, 119–20, 264,
    268
    emotional and social development
    252–4
    growth 235, 240–1
    intellectual development 249
    physical development 244
    smoking 195
    voluntary services for 70
    working with 94
oral presentations 2, 34–6, 46
organisations 53, 149–50, 223–5,
    227, 292–3
osteopathy 65
overcrowding, and health 181

P
paediatric community team 102–3
PAMS see Professions Allied to
    Medicine
parenthood, and smoking 195
patients, needs of 45
Patients Charter 127–9, 138
patients' records 117, 124–5
PCGs see Primary Care Groups
peak flow meters 215–17
perception 246
Personal Health Records 237
personal hygiene 204–5
personal organisation 2, 5–7
personal qualities, and jobs 87, 89,
    97, 100
PHCT see Primary Health Care Team
physical contact 115–15
physical health 161, 162–4
    indicators 210, 211–20
    stress 161, 162–4
placements 41–6
planning and prioritising tasks 22–3
play group 98
policies, for staff 127
pollution, and personal development
    268–9
portfolio, compiling 2, 8–9, 10
poverty 177, 182–3, 267, 270
PQ4R 14
practice staff 60, 99–100
pregnancy 171–2, 192, 195, 283
prejudice 120
presentation skills (written
    assignments) 26–7
    see also oral presentations
previewing 14
Primary Care Groups 57, 59–60, 64,
    75
Primary Health Care Team 60, 75,
    101
Princess Royal Trust 76
private services 54, 55, 94
    alternative therapists 65
    fostering and adoption agencies
    106
    health insurance 267
    home care 69
    nurseries 106
    residential homes 69, 106
    Walk In Centres 64
Professions Allied to Medicine 99
projects 2, 8, 16–28
proof-reading 25–6
proteins 165, 166–9, 170
psycho-social theory 252, 253

puberty 238–9
    emotional and social development
        251–2
    growth 235, 238–9
    intellectual development 248–9
    physical development 244
pulse rate 217–20

Q
qualifications 9
questioning 15

R
Race Relations Act (1976) 119
racial discrimination 266
radiographers 99
radiotherapists 99
reading 2, 9–10, 12, 15
reasoning 246
receptionists 100
receptive reading 12
reciting 15
records of achievement 9, 41
reflecting back (listening skill) 111–12
reflective reading 12, 15
refuges, for children 106
Regional Health Authorities 57
regions, NHS 55–7
registered child minder 98
rehabilitation 67
religious beliefs, respecting 136–7
religious groups, discrimination 118
residential care 67, 94, 96, 105–6,
        125–6, 128
resources 51–3, 148–50, 223–7, 291–
        293
respite care 67
review, importance of 15, 30–1
rights, supporting people's 125–36
Royal National Institute for the Deaf
        140

S
salt, dangers of in diet 200
sanitation, and health 181
scanning 12
scattergrams 217
schools 94, 102
Secondary Care 60, 64, 75, 104

Secretary of State of Health 55
secure accommodation 106
self-appraisal 44–5, 46
self-concept 270–3
self-esteem 36, 249, 252, 254, 262–3,
        273
self-image 249
Sex Discrimination Act (1975) 119
Sexual Health Clinic 207
sexuality
    discrimination 266
    safe sex 206, 207, 208
    secondary characteristics 238
    sexual behaviour 206–8
    sexually transmitted diseases
        206–8
signing alphabet 140
skills checklist (work experience
        placements) 44
skimming 12
sleep and behaviour clinics 102
smoking 178, 194–6, 270
social care
    jobs 84–6, 94–8
    statutory services 65–7
social class, and health 177–9
social development 234
social disengagement theory 252, 253
social exclusion 267
social factors, in personal development
        254–68
social health 161, 162–4, 210
Social Services
    client groups 67, 95
    Code of Practice 126
    early years 104
    modernising 67
    organisational chart 66, 95
    services provided by 67
    working for 94
socialisation 254, 264
sociologists 261
software 46, 52, 227
speech therapists 99, 102
spell-checkers 24, 25
spider diagrams 19, 20
Standards of Care 129
statutory services 54, 55, 65–7, 104
stereotypes 120, 264, 266

stress, and health 201–4
Stroke Association 144
study skills 1–53, 15
suicide 257, 258, 266
support, types of 274–83, 281–2
surgical care 64

T
TB 181
teams, working in 37–40
teenage pregnancy 184
Tertiary Care 60, 75
tests, timed 29–34
therapists, alternative 65
time-planning 2, 5–8
toddlers clubs 107

U
unemployment, and health 180, 183
United Kingdom Central Council for
        Nursing, Midwifery and Health
Code of Practice 123, 126

V
Venereal Disease Clinic 207
vitamins 165, 166–7, 172
voluntary services 54, 55, 69–75, 70,
        71–3, 74–5, 106, 107

W
wants versus needs 258–60, 270
water, in diet 165, 167
weight 212–13, 214–15, 236, 238
work-experience 2, 41–6
working collaboratively 2, 16, 37–40
working conditions, and health 177
workplaces 41–2
unsafe practices in 208–10
World Health Organisation 160–2,
        210–11
writing skills 23–5

Y
young people 94, 191–2, 194, 195,
        205
see also adolescence
youth and community work 94
'youth culture' 265